# AROMATHERAPY
# Scent
## AND
# Psyche

# AROMATHERAPY
# Scent
## AND
# Psyche

## USING ESSENTIAL OILS FOR
## PSYCHOLOGICAL AND PHYSICAL
## WELL-BEING

## Peter & Kate Damian

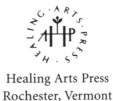

Healing Arts Press
Rochester, Vermont

Healing Arts Press
One Park Street
Rochester, Vermont 05767
www.gotoit.com

*Note to the reader: This book is intended as an informational guide. The remedies, approaches, and techniques described herein are meant to supplement, and not to be a substitute for, professional medical care or treatment. They should not be used to treat a serious ailment without prior consultation with a qualified health care professional.*

Library of Congress Cataloging-in-Publication Data
Damian, Peter.
      Aromatherapy : scent and psyche : using essential oils for
physical and emotional well-being / Peter and Kate Damian.
          p. cm.
      Includes bibliographical references and index.
      ISBN 0-89281-530-2
      1. Aromatherapy—Popular works.   I. Damian, Kate.   II. Title.
RM666.A68D35    1995
615'.321—dc20                                                        95–15998
                                                                              CIP

Printed and bound in the United States

10 9 8 7 6 5 4 3

Healing Arts Press is a division of Inner Traditions International

Distributed to the book trade in Canada by Publishers Group West (PGW),
Toronto, Ontario
Distributed to the health food trade in Canada by Alive Books,
Toronto and Vancouver
Distributed to the book trade in the United Kingdom by Deep Books, London
Distributed to the book trade in Australia by Millennium Books, Newtown, N. S. W.
Distributed to the book trade in New Zealand by Tandem Press, Auckland
Distributed to the book trade in South Africa by
Alternative Books, Ferndale

*To our parents*

# Contents

Acknowledgments      ix

Chapter One      1
    Introduction to Aromatherapy

Chapter Two      33
    Phytoaromatherapy and the Theory
    of Disease

Chapter Three      56
    Smell and the Psychology of Scent

Chapter Four      108
    Aromatherapy Today and Tomorrow: Theory
    and Practice, Issues and Debates

Chapter Five      141
    Psychotherapeutic Effects of Essential Oils

Chapter Six      166
    The Chemistry of Essential Oils

Chapter Seven      179
    Essential Oil Profiles

Appendix      209
    Floral Waters In Aromatherapy
    Aromatic Diffusors
    Basic Principles of Essential Oil Blending

Charts and Tables                                              211
    Aromatherapy Usage Guide
    Chakra Oil Blending Guide
    Essential Oil Quick Reference Table
    Essential Oil Repertory
Selected Bibliography                                          233
Aromatherapy Essential Oil Companies                          235
Index                                                          237

# Acknowledgments

We express our sincere gratitude and appreciation to friends and associates whose brilliant work and pioneering efforts in the field of phytoaromatherapy have been inspirational; especially Robert Tisserand, Marcel Lavabre, Kurt Schnaubelt, Annemarie Buhler, Dr. Jean-Claude Lapraz, and Dr. Daniel Penoel.

# 1

# Introduction To Aromatherapy

## DEFINITIONS, EXPLANATIONS, FEATURES

Aromatherapy is a modern term for what are actually various therapeutic and aesthetic uses made of derivatives or extracts from a wide variety of plants. More precisely, aromatherapy is the specific use of *pure essential oils* by topical (skin) application or inhalation. A pure essential oil is the condensation of a plant's vital "essence"—the soul of the plant—in which is stored vital solar energy. This essential oil is what gives the plant its fragrance. It is also where the plant's most valuable therapeutic and nutritional properties are highly concentrated. The essence is produced by special cells within the plant and contains, among other things, phytohormones: "chemical messengers" that, like human hormones, transmit cellular information throughout the body in response to stress and environmental conditions. The essence or essential oil protects the plant from disease, parasites, and other would-be predators, while attracting certain insects for reproductive pollination. In some cases, essential oils act as selective weed-killers, allowing the plant to establish its territory by eliminating competitive vegetation. In harsh desert climates, myrrh and frankincense actually emit essential oil vapors to shield themselves from extreme sunlight.

The vital essences of plants are converted into pure essential oils and aromatic hydrosols (floral waters) by the mechanical process of steam distillation. Only after extraction by the production method of distillation does an essence become an essential oil. Although we generally use the term *essential oil* to describe all the oils employed by aromatherapy, those

1

that are extracted by other methods are not precisely pure essential oils. For example, oils extracted by expression (cold pressing or pressure) retain more of the plant's essence. Some plants (e.g., jasmine) will not release their oil unless a solvent is used. Oils obtained by such processes involving chemical solvents are called *concrétes* or *absolutes*. These and other production methods will be explained in chapter 6. For now it is enough to know that essential oils can be extracted from certain trees, shrubs, herbs, flowers, and grasses, wherein they may be found in virtually any part of the plant: seeds, flowers, fruit, leaves, stalks and stems, roots, bark, wood, needles, and resins.

The proportional yield of essential oil from plants will vary from a small fraction of 1 percent to as much as 10 percent. The process can be slow, laborious, and quite expensive. It takes 500 pounds of sage or rosemary to make a quart of oil; a ton of thyme will yield less than a quart. It may take thousands of pounds of rose petals to solvent-extract a pound of rose oil. More than 8 million hand-picked jasmine blossoms may produce a mere kilogram (2.2 pounds) of essential oil. (Jasmine and rose are two of the most costly essential oils.) The amount of plant material and the production time required—or allowed—to produce an essential oil will affect its cost and quality. Slow-distilling 1 kilogram of oil from 1,000 kilograms of prime-picked flowers will add to the cost of the oil as well as to the higher-quality concentration of its therapeutic and nutritional constituents and properties.

Most essential oils are colorless or pale yellow; some (e.g., German or blue chamomile) are deeply pigmented. The majority of colored oils (e.g., bergamot and jasmine) are either essences or absolutes. Although highly concentrated, essential oils are not oily. Lighter than water (with a few exceptions), they are usually highly fluid. That they are lipid (fat) soluble rather than water soluble is an important attribute that allows their easier, faster, deeper, and more thorough penetration into the skin. (Since the skin is waterproof, water-soluble substances are resisted.) The rapid skin absorbency of essential oils is also partly due to their highly volatile (evaporative) nature. The characteristics of essential oil molecules allow their ready passage into the bloodstream. Because of their volatility, essential oils are best packaged in airtight aluminum or amber glass containers, which should also be kept in cool, dark, dry storage.

A more inclusive term, *phytotherapy*—"plant therapy," or plant medicine—better describes the varied treatment applications using plant extracts and materials other than, and including, essential oils. Phytotherapy incorporates the internal use of essential oils, principally by ingestion. The term *phytotherapy* is often combined with, or used interchangeably for, *aromatherapy*. However, it is just as applicable as a synonym for *herbalism* or *herbology*.

Additional methods of extraction that do not produce essential oils, such as the creation of tinctures or liniments, are included in phytotherapy. Two others are decoction (boiling of leaves or roots to gain an extract) and infusion (pouring hot water over herbs or flowers, then briefly steeping them much as one makes tea). Likewise, an infusion oil can be created by soaking aromatic plant material in vegetable oil, thereby infusing the oil with the plant's fragrance. This is an ancient technique in the practice of *aromatics.*

Aromatics is the aesthetic or therapeutic use of scents and fragrances that are derived from plants but are not necessarily essential oils. Ancient aromatherapy practiced prior to the discovery or general implementation of distillation (and therefore of pure essential oils) is more appropriately considered aromatics. Aromatics ought not be confused with simple perfumery involving fragrances that largely contain synthetic oils or scents diluted in alcohol and water, which merely smell pleasant or mask other odors. Personal anointment with infused oils was understood to provide genuine health benefits as well as aesthetic appeal and, moreover, to confer protection from contagious disease, owing in part to the antimicrobial powers of the natural botanical ingredients.

## HISTORICAL OVERVIEW

Although the term *aromatherapy* has been in use for less than a century, the therapeutic, spiritual (religious and liturgical), and cosmetic uses of aromatic oils have at least a 5,000-year history. Phytotherapy or herbology has surely been practiced even longer. The spread of aromatherapy (aromatics, phytotherapy) has followed the westward course of civilization, beginning in the oriental cultures of China, India, Persia, and Egypt. The earliest scriptures of the Hindu religion—the Vedas—mention several hundred perfumes and aromatic products, codifying them for both liturgical and therapeutic practices. This knowledge has been maintained for at least 3,000 years through the Indian practice of Ayurvedic medicine, in which many of the essential oils used in aromatherapy have been a useful part. A principal feature of Ayurvedic medicine is aromatic massage using infused oils made from indigenous herbs and woods. The ancient Chinese also advocated massage. The oldest surviving medical texts from China, each dating back to c. 2700 B.C., are classics of herbal medicine. It is very likely that the ancient civilizations of China and India were practicing some form of aromatics as well as phytotherapy while such practices were occurring in Egypt, about which we know considerably more.

## The Middle East

As long ago as 3000 B.C., the Egyptians were utilizing plants for medicine, massage therapy, surgery, food preparation and preservation, religious rituals, and mummification. Since steam distillation had not yet been developed, they prepared aromatic oils and incense by soaking plant materials in base oils or fats. There is some evidence that later Egyptians experimented with crude methods of distillation. Zozime, a third-century chemist, reported designs for stills that he observed on a temple wall in Memphis.

Hundreds of plants contain high levels of antibacterial, antiviral, antifungal, and otherwise antiseptic constituents. The awareness of these properties of plant substances prompted their use in food preparation and preservation, and in mummification. During the thousands of years before refrigeration, people from India to Europe were using herbs and oils to preserve meats and to make them more digestible. This tradition endures in the culinary arts by the use of herbs, spices, and condiments to improve digestion, both by their stimulation of digestive processes and by their direct catalytic and antiseptic action upon meat. (Today, 50 percent of the world's essential oil production is for the food industry's use of flavorings; about 5 percent is for aromatherapy, a small but significant and increasing figure.) The Egyptians likewise embalmed their pharaohs in essential oils to kill and inhibit bacteria and thus limit decomposition. It is worth repeating that unlike synthetic perfumes or commercial aerosols and deodorants, the fragrance of an essential oil does not merely mask foul odors arising from putrefaction or infections; it actually suppresses them by a physicochemical action that destroys, hinders, or neutralizes germs.

In early Mesopotamia, the Sumerians, Babylonians, Hebrews and other ancient Semitic peoples also utilized aromatics (oils and incense) for religious purposes. Ancient spiritual healing and religious or liturgical practices in which aromatic oils and plants were used to expand consciousness and improve meditation should be viewed as the first applications of aromapsychology. Such practices naturally accomplished what modern medical science has attempted through the manufacturing and prescription of mood-altering drugs, hallucinogens, and other kinds of synthetic chemicals intended to improve physical or mental performance or otherwise alter and control human behavior. The aromatic fumigations and incense burning done to dispel various miasmic conditions—not just foul spirits—and purify the atmosphere are equivalent to the later use of disinfectant aerosols, atomizers, and humidifiers to cleanse and condition the air. Today's psychologists are just now beginning to reconsider the more intelligent and safer prescription of natural mood-enhancing substances, among which none are better than essential oils.

## The Greeks and Romans

The ancient Greeks were perhaps the first to distinguish those psychological disorders arising from organic causes from others of a supernatural or metaphysical origin. Mental illness was often diagnosed as a disorganization of temperament or imbalance of the humours, treatable by herbs, aromatics, or other natural means. The Greeks' appreciation of aromatics and essential oils, although spiritual, was more systematically applied in medicine and also in warfare to stimulate aggression and to heal battle wounds. Like many Greek practices and traditions, these were passed on to the Romans. Dioscorides, a first-century Greek surgeon in the Roman army of Nero, included a chapter on oils in his medical encyclopedia, which remained a standard medical text for more than a thousand years. He too made early experiments with the crude distillation of the "quintessence" of plants, producing camphor and turpentine. Both before and after Dioscorides, Greek physicians such as Hippocrates and Asclepiades utilized aromatics. Hippocrates successfully combated plagues by fumigating the entire city of Athens with aromatic substances, a practice repeated somewhat less systematically centuries later in Europe during its notorious plagues and epidemics. In the nineteenth century, when perfumes were made with real, natural botanical fragrances, perfumery workers were virtually immune to the cholera outbreaks of the time.

Like the earlier Greeks and Romans, the eighth-century Arabs carried their knowledge of medicinal plants throughout Asia Minor, the Middle

East, and by further invasions of Europe and North Africa. Later eleventh-century Christian Crusaders returned to Europe with much knowledge of the famous perfumes of Arabia as well as of alchemy, the forerunner of modern chemistry. These events continued the extensive trade in odoriferous plants already begun and which had spread from India throughout the Greek and Roman empires.

## Avicenna

The invention of distillation is attributed to the Persians, particularly to the renowned physician, philosopher, and alchemist Hakim Abu Ali Abdulah Husayn Ibn Sina, known more familiarly in the West as Avicenna. Actually, some perfumed waters produced by primitive distillation had been used in Persia prior to Avicenna's birth, and by the thirteenth century the famous Damascan rose water was being exported as far away as China, India, and Europe to be used for a variety of purposes. It seems, therefore, more likely that distillation, which produces both floral waters (aromatic hydrosols) and pure essential oils, was invented and developed over a century and was later perfected by Avicenna for the specific production of essential oils. Arabic manuscripts from his day show drawings of stills, the basic principles of which remain the same today despite modern advancements in design technology. The invention of distillation led to the discovery and production of alcohol. Alcohol and essential oils made the production of non-oily perfumes possible.

Despite Avicenna's breakthrough, distillation remained, at least until the Middle Ages, primarily a means for preparing floral waters rather than essential oils. Evidently, whenever the process resulted in the precipitation of essential oil, such as the crystallization of rose oil on the surface of rose water (which was apparently Avicenna's first successful experiment), the oil was more often regarded as an unwanted by-product than as a new and desirable one.

Born in A.D. 980 in what is now Uzbekistan, Avicenna displayed his extraordinary intelligence at a very early age. A child prodigy, whose genius was nurtured by his learned father, Avicenna was appointed chief physician of the royal court at age fourteen. His father's death and local political upheaval drove Avicenna into a life of wandering that led him to Persia, where he found refuge and gained the patronage of Persian royalty.

Despite his brief lifetime (he died in 1037), Avicenna authored some 276 works, most in a series of volumes, dealing with an enormous scope of subjects ranging from science to religion, mathematics to music, and including astrology, history, and economics. Yet, his well-deserved fame as "Prince of Physicians" stands upon one work: *Al-Qanun fi'l Tibb* (*The Canon of Medicine*), which is highly regarded as one of the most famous, important, and influential books of medicine in the history of both East and West. Arranged in five volumes, the *Canon* summarized all the known medical knowledge of the civilized world, including that of the Greeks, Europeans, Persians, Arabs, Indians, and Chinese. Translated into nearly every language of the Western world, it became a standard text for 500 years and the basis for most medieval schools of medicine, and it remains the manual for all practitioners of the Tibb tradition that Avicenna founded. The traditional medicine of Islam, Tibb is the treatment for more than 1 billion Moslem and non-Moslem people worldwide. From an Arabic word meaning "medicine of the physical, mental, and spiritual realms," Tibb is based on two concepts: the Doctrine of Naturals, establishing normal standards for the human body by which disease is surmised from contrasting abnormalities; and the Doctrine of Causes, which identifies and explains the origins of those abnormalities. Primary symptoms are considered signs indicating the imbalance or "intemperament" that allows the disease to first occur.

Implementing his system of therapeutics, Avicenna established hospitals and advanced the processes of filtration, sublimation, and calcination, which are indispensable to the distillation of pure essential oils. Besides imparting his knowledge of dietetics, Avicenna systemized methods of urinalysis, pulse diagnosis, spinal manipulations, and traction for broken limbs, and he assembled an extensive pharmacology of more than 800 plant substances and their effects upon the body.

## Europe

The tenth-century rise of European exploration and crusades, and repeated Moslem invasions before and after that time, brought knowledge of distillation into Western Europe. The first reliable description of distillation of real essential oils is ascribed to a thirteenth-century Catalan physician, Arnald de Villanova, who apparently introduced the art of distillation to standard European medical practice. Nevertheless, there is some evidence suggesting that distillation specifically of essential oils (not floral waters, a specialty of medieval and postmedieval pharmacies) may not have come into general use until as late as the sixteenth century. Meanwhile, the great fifteenth-century European explorers had been continually arriving with many new plants and aromas gathered from around the world.

The sixteenth century brought the next major advance in aromatherapy and the production of pure essential oils. In an era when fragrances, perfumes, floral waters, and herbs were in wide popular usage, a German physician, Hieronymous Brunschweig (also known as Jerome of Brunswick), between the years 1500 and 1507 wrote a two-volume book on the distillation process. In it he describes all techniques and products of distillation, specifically mentioning four essential oils. His last great work was published much later in the century and expanded references to twenty-five essential oils. Between those dates and throughout the century, many equally important written contributions to the knowledge of distillation and essential oils were made by Swiss, German, French, and Italian physicians and alchemists, such as Conrad Gesner, Walter Ryff, Adam Lonicer, Valerius Cordus, Joseph Du Chesne, and Giovanni Battista della Porta.

The seventeenth century is considered the grand era of English herbalists, most notably Nicholas Culpeper, John Gerard, and John Parkinson, whose phytotherapy included a small representation of essential oils. Yet, in the seventeenth and eighteenth centuries, it was chiefly the European pharmacists or apothecaries, too numerous to name, especially in France and Germany, who contributed most to the emergence of modern aromatherapy by their improved methods of distillation and investigation of the nature and value of essential oils. Although by the eighteenth century nearly every herbalist and many physicians used essential oils, phytotherapy was to receive a major setback from the advent of chemistry. Ironically, it would be the earlier alchemists, with renewed enthusiasm for the use of chemicals discovered in their laboratories as drugs (an idea initiated centuries before by the alchemist Paracelsus), who would inspire the gradual rift, starting about 1650, between physicians who increasingly favored chemical drugs and those who remained faithful to phytotherapy. More and more eighteenth-century and then nineteenth-century chemists attempted to isolate the constituents of plants for drugs rather than using the plant itself. The word *drug* derives from the old Dutch word for "dry," as in the drying of herbs for medicinal purposes. While chemical analyses of herbs brought us aspirin (from willow bark) and atropine (from belladonna)—indeed, most medicines have been developed in one way or another from the study of plants—regrettably, the trend of drug development and therapy, leading to today's pharmaceutical industry and its dangerous synthetic chemical products, has also had dire consequences.

After technological improvements allowed scientists to view microorganisms, an etiological school of thought emerged in the late nineteenth century that asserted the bacteriological cause of disease. Before then, all physicians, basing their assumptions principally upon the works of Avicenna and the early Greek masters (Galen, Dioscorides, and Hippocrates), believed that disease arose as evidence of organic malfunction. This idea was rejected by the bacteriologists, who claimed that a specific microbe or virus was responsible for each disease and its symptoms or lesions. A century earlier, biologists had concluded that because they couldn't isolate and quantify the four humours (elemental substances) that were central to the traditional theory of disease linking the medical systems of Avicenna and the Greeks, the theory must be inherently flawed. By the end of the nineteenth century, the bacteriological school of thought had undermined and would thereafter supplant the nearly 800-year influence of Tibb medicine upon European thought. The search for microbial and other microscopic causes of disease, and for the drugs and vaccines to combat them, became and largely remains the preoccupation of modern medical science.

Like their modern successors, the great naturopathic and holistic physicians of the past, while acknowledging the existence of bacteria and viruses, do not consider microorganisms to be the primary cause of disease. Instead, they view them as opportunistic invaders exploiting a disordered metabolism or organic malfunction of the human body. In their opinion, there is no single, specific cause of disease; each unhealthy condition arises from various factors usually occurring in combination. "A microbe is not always the cause of an illness," writes Dr. Jean Valnet, an eminent French physician and a modern pioneer in the field of aromatherapy. "Normally it simply bears witness to a deficiency in the organism under attack." The presence of a microbe is less important than the constitutional health of the host, adds Valnet. "Infection does not automatically follow the penetration of an organism by a microbe, the germ has to find a suitable breeding-ground." This is apparent from the plain observation that not every person exposed to or even found harboring a particular microbe will become ill; natural healthy resistance or immunity prevents it. Disease cannot take hold in an otherwise healthy organism. Therefore, it becomes most important to treat the patient and not the disease, which is precisely what all naturopathic and holistic systems, including aromatherapy, intend to do. They treat the cause, not the symptoms.

Still, the advent of the microbial theory of disease provided yet another opportunity to demonstrate the effective versatility of essential oils in combating illness. Although the use of essential oils would eventually fall out of favor among physicians smitten by the allure of drugs, the first successful laboratory tests demonstrating the antibacterial properties of essential oils were also conducted in the late nineteenth century. They were prompted by the observation that tuberculosis cases in the flower-growing districts of France were uncommonly rare. Indeed, French workers who processed fragrant flowers and herbs remained virtually free of any respiratory ailments. (This is highly reminiscent of reports made about the nineteenth-century perfume workers and their resistance to cholera. The same conclusions ought to be drawn.) Subsequent French studies similarly showed that the microorganisms of yellow fever and glanders (a contagious horse disease) were readily killed by essential oils. Since then, countless tests and experiments have demonstrated the antimicrobial or antiseptic powers of essential oils, frequently against diphtheria and tuberculosis. Nevertheless, the use of essential oils in medicinal preparations or as medicinal agents became subordinate to their employment in the production of perfumes, beverages, and foodstuffs. By the mid-twentieth century, their pharmaceutical application had been reduced to little more than flavoring agents for chemical drugs. At that point, modern aromatherapy owed much of its survival to the food and fragrance industries, which continued research and experimentation with essential oils, and also to those great late nineteenth-century and early twentieth-century chemists whose systematic study of essential oils led to the elucidation and analysis of their molecular structure and chemical components. The discovery of active essential oil chemical constituents has brought about new understandings and, of course, new controversies. Predictably, as newly revealed components were first identified, synthesized, and then commercially manufactured, a new industry of synthetic and isolated aromatics was born.

## Aromathérapie

The revival of aromatherapy began in the late 1920s with a French cosmetic chemist named René-Maurice Gattefossé. It was he who coined the term *aromathérapie*—aromatherapy—which became the title of his first book. Gattefossé's fascination with essential oils commenced with personal observations he made while working for his family's perfumery. He noted that many of the essential oils used in the perfume products were superior antiseptics to the chemical antiseptics that were added. He was particularly impressed by the extraordinary healing effectiveness of lavender when, after burning his hand during a lab explosion, he immediately immersed the injured hand in pure lavender oil. The hand not only healed within a few hours but it did so without infection or scarring. This motivated his first exploration into the uses of essential oils for dermatology and cosmetics. From there, Gattefossé viewed the enormous potential and great possibilities in aromatherapy research.

Soon thereafter, another Frenchman, Albert Couvreur, published his book on the medical application of essential oils. Simultaneously, other research began appearing independently from around the world. In Australia, the antiseptic and antimicrobial benefits of tea tree oil were being displayed and chronicled by another chemist, A.R. Penfold, while in Italy, Giovanni Gatti and Renato Cajola were investigating the psychological effects of essential oils. Like many other things, the progress of aromatherapy stalled during World War II, but even under those difficult circumstances the torch was being carried by Dr. Jean Valnet, who while an army surgeon utilized what he had learned from Gattefossé's work to treat soldiers wounded on the battlefield. Valnet continued his medical practice after the war, incorporating essential oils into every phase. His definitive book, *The Practice of Aromatherapy*, was later published in 1964 and is now available in English. Thanks largely to Dr. Valnet's instruction of other physicians, there are now several establishments in France serving the need for education in aromatherapy and more than 1,500 physicians who prescribe essential oils.

One of Valnet's students, a French biochemist, Marguerite Maury, contributed a more personalized, holistic vision of aromatherapy that reemphasized the external use of essential oils in massage. Just three years before her death, her ideas were published in one of her two books, *The Secret of Life and Youth*, recently translated into English. In it Maury revives the ancient traditional philosophies of medicine that include aromatic massage, and she proposes the concept of an "individualized prescription"—a blend of essential oils that would harmonize the physical, psychological (mental/emotional), and spiritual nature of the patient, thereby balancing and normalizing the whole person. By eschewing the *in vitro* perspective of essential oils that accentuates their internal use, Maury represents a truer expression of aromatherapy as defined earlier.

The list of significant figures in modern aromatherapy has grown over the past thirty years to include Professor Paolo Rovesti of the University of Milan, who advanced the psychological research of Gatti and Cajola; Micheline Arcier and Daniele Ryman, the former a student of Valnet and both disciples of Marguerite Maury, who like their mentor have expanded interest in aromatherapy into Great Britain; and medical doctors Paul Belaiche, Daniel Penoel, and Jean-Claude Lapraz. Other contributions come from the chemist Pierre Franchomme, as well as from British massage therapists Robert Tisserand, Shirley Price, and Patricia Davis, whose work and writings have greatly popularized aromatherapy not only in England but in the United States. These are but a few of the more recognizable names; there are many less publicized but equally important individuals whose accomplishments and contributions in and to aromatherapy are far too plentiful to enumerate.

# FIELDS OF APPLICATION

Human development and the advances of the past century have coupled with the rich potential and amazing versatility of aromatherapy and pure essential oils to greatly widen their application. These various traditional and modern applications are broadly categorized as clinical/medical, aesthetic/cosmetic, and holistic/naturopathic, or sometimes according to the administration method of essential oils: internally (ingestion), externally (topical), or aromatically (inhalation). Since essential oils have simultaneous physical and psychological affects, and human response to them will, therefore, occur physically, emotionally, and mentally as well as spiritually, separate categories cannot always be maintained by sharp lines of theory or hard barriers of practice. Aromatherapy and essential oils will invariably give crossover results and reciprocal benefits.

# Medicine

One clinical/medical application of essential oils is as an alternative to chemical synthetic drugs, not only as antimicrobials but as mood-enhancing agents useful in psychology or psychiatry. In *The Practice of Aromatherapy*, Dr. Valnet offers a sure definition of safe and healthful treatment: "any substance or process that is non-toxic and constant in its effects when faced with the same symptoms." By his criterion, essential oils are certainly safe, healthful, and effective, whereas modern chemically synthesized drugs too often are not. A century of research and evaluation has confirmed that essential oils are effective antimicrobial agents and that they are without the unpleasant side-effects associated with medical antibiotics. Essential oils have a profound influence on virtually every physiological system, process, and function. They assist the elimination of toxins at the cellular level and are antimicrobial and antiseptic not only by their direct activity but by strengthening the body's own immune system. Unlike synthetic drugs, essential oils prescribed for physical or psychological ills do not harmfully or indiscriminately impose their action upon the body but instead help the body to help itself. They do not attack or weaken the organism while attacking the disease. They have a natural suitability that, unlike medical antibiotics, counters infectious germs while sparing—even promoting— useful, beneficial microorganisms.

Conversely, "Antibiotics act by modifying the chemical constitution of the microbes, so that the antibodies the organism produces for its own defense will be effective only against a modified germ," writes Dr. Valnet. "They are, therefore, only 'false antibodies' impotent against the real agent of infection, the germ in its original state." Frequent use builds an escalating tolerance requiring increased dosages because microorganisms adapt to the antibiotics faster than does the body. In short, microorganisms build a resistance to antibiotics. Hence, antibiotics become increasingly less efficient and more a threat to the organism than they are to the infectious germs. Their short-term results may cause secondary infections or lead later to more advanced and more resistant infections. (The problem of tolerance also occurs with the administration of chemically synthesized narcotics, tranquilizers, and the like, to which the organism becomes gradually habituated, requiring either increasingly larger dosages or frequent changes of medication. As Valnet says, "Accustomed to reacting to the different things that attack it, the body will become habituated to everything that is in any way adulterated, harmful, or toxic.") Microbes build little or no resistance to essential oils, perhaps because essential oils are the natural defense mechanism of the plant, and their chemical complexity, which defies scientific analysis, also confounds and thwarts would-be invaders.

The deleterious effects of drugs involve more than tolerance, adaptation, and addiction. Drugs place severe stresses upon all physiological systems, instigating numerous biochemical, glandular, and nutritional imbalances and deficiencies. No drug listed in the *Physicians' Desk Reference* is without some side-effects that may sicken or disable the patient or worse— these drugs include antibiotics, antihistamines, barbituates, tranquilizers, steroids and hormones, contraceptives, painkillers, and heart medicines. Like many physicians, Dr. Valnet suggests that drugs be regarded as crisis or emergency remedies rather than as first-choice medicines: "But if it is logical, and in truth essential, to take risks inherent in their use when the severity of the condition justifies it, the disadvantages of these medicaments must surely forbid their being administered systematically or lightly for illnesses susceptible enough to less dangerous treatments." Aromatherapy and essential oils offer physicians a safe and effective alternative for nearly any condition that might otherwise indicate the use of drugs. That is not to suggest that aromatherapy is a cure-all (no system or therapy is) or that essential oils are entirely without hazards. As we shall learn in subsequent chapters about the safe use of essential oils, some oils require cautious and discretionary use, but the potential toxicity and hazards of essential oils are mild and minimal in comparison with drugs.

The clinical/medical use of essential oils also includes them in anal or vaginal suppositories, in topical applications for dermatological conditions, and in germicidal sprays or aerosols. As observed by Dr. H. Sztark, French medical inspector of schools in the late 1930s, "Being both volatile and antiseptic, essential oils are the ideal means of preventing the spread of airborne infection." The inhalation or topical administration of essential oils has decided advantages over their internal use, especially when combined with other therapies such as massage. They seem to be better absorbed through the skin and nose, and their effects are more immediate. By either means, essential oils gain easy and unaltered entry into the bloodstream as they are taken up by the capillaries and lymph ducts (when applied topically) or the lungs (when inhaled); they are initially unchanged by the liver metabolism that occurs when they are swallowed.

## Massage

The historically synergetic relationship between massage and aromatherapy extends back to the ancient Indians and Chinese, who like Asclepiades and Marguerite Maury, were strong advocates of aromatic massage. Avicenna, too, recommended the benefits of the "restorative friction" of massage for a variety of purposes and included oils, perfumed ointments, and calefacient (warming) medicines in the process. The many therapeutic results of massage upon the circulatory system, lymphatic system, muscles, organs, and glands have been well documented and scientifically proved; combined with essential oils they are greatly enhanced and expanded. The healthful vegetable oils used in massage, which are also lipid soluble and therefore absorbed into the skin, make excellent carriers for essential oils. The effects are threefold: The topical application of essential oils restores, rejuvenates, and nourishes the skin, something that is also accomplished when essential oils are included in aesthetic/cosmetic treatments. The essential oils assist the massage effects that liberate toxins from muscles, open congested nerves, and increase blood and lymph flow. Meanwhile, the oils are also released aromatically and taken up by the olfactory systems of the nose.

In summary, aromatic massage will (1) enliven and tone the skin and the subcutaneous and connective tissues, increasing circulation and thus facilitating the removal of toxins while assisting skin nutrition; (2) reduce or eliminate conditions of lymphatic stasis, edema, and inflammation; (3) stimulate muscle irrigation (releasing toxic buildup such as lactic acid) and restore muscle tone, thus reducing fatigue and accelerating recuperation; (4) harmonize or balance the autonomic nervous system and cerebrospinal system; (5) tone and normalize the visceral digestive organs; and (6) normalize functions of the endocrine glands. Although aromatic massage is generally recognized as the most complete and comprehensive body therapy, other bodywork systems, such as shiatsu, reflexology, acupressure, and polarity therapy, can also greatly benefit from the incorporation of essential oils.

## Cosmetology

Clearly, the superior advantage to skin care provided by aromatherapy is the capacity of essential oils to advance cellular renewal through increased circulation, hydration, and waste removal. In this way, the essential oils also

15

exhibit their natural "homeostatic intelligence" by regulating the skin's sebaceous secretions according to its requirements, just as they do for glands elsewhere in the body. Essential oils will invigorate a hypoactive organ or stabilize one that is hyperactive, thereby restoring homeostasis. Once an essential oil is applied topically, it needs approximately 20 to 90 minutes to be entirely absorbed into the body. Excess body fat will slow absorption, as will edema, sluggish circulation, and excessive tissue toxication. Since essential oils are immiscible in water, oil absorption will be diminished by sweating. The stronger the blood circulation, the faster and more thoroughly the essential oils are absorbed. Essential oils are excreted from a healthy body within 3 to 6 hours after treatment, perhaps three times as long from an unhealthy body.

Aromatherapy is becoming big business for health and beauty spas, salons, and the cosmetic and fragrance industries, whose advertising approach touts the benefits of essential oils applied topically as well as their aromatic effects. They are marketing not only hair, face, and body products but also room fresheners and mood enhancers. Some of these companies are using true essential oils; others are not. Rather broad interpretations and vague use of terms like "pure," "organic," and "natural" permit wide latitude in market advertising. It is a fundamental precept of aromatherapy that genuine results are achieved only by pure essential oils. This excludes synthetics, perfumes, and aromatic chemicals. Fragrance companies like to argue that there is no difference between synthetics and naturals and that because of widespread adulteration pure essential oils are virtually nonexistent. Quality determinants, and the real and important distinctions between natural and synthetic oils, are discussed in another chapter. Suffice it to say for now that aromatherapists rightly reply that there is indeed a significant difference: as an organic substance, a pure  or natural essential oil contains at least several hundred components (most unidentified or undiscovered) that work synergetically and holistically,  making the oils safer, more effective, and impossible to replicate. Natural rose oil, for example, may have as many as 2,000 components; synthetic rose oil might have fifty. It is precisely an essential oil's complexity that provides its many benefits and effects. Lavender, the most versatile pure essential oil, counters stress, depression, and fatigue; lowers blood pressure and soothes heart palpitations; relieves aches and pains; heals burns; calms nerves; is anti-inflammatory and antiseptic; and is an insect repellent and a remedy for menstrual difficulties—among other things. Synthetic lavender?

## Psychology

Everyone seems to agree that scents have a remarkable influence upon the human organism. Although the mechanisms and processes of olfaction remain largely mysterious, science's progressive knowledge and understanding of our sense of smell opens exciting new vistas and possibilities for aromatherapy research. Although more limited in range than sight or hearing (you can see or hear something at a longer distance than you can smell it) our sense of smell is estimated to be 10,000 times more acute than our other senses and sensitive to some 10,000 chemical compounds. Once registered, scent stimuli travel more quickly to the brain than do either sight or sound; how this happens is still a matter for some speculation. Olfactory responses to odors induce the brain, or at least parts of it, to stimulate the release of hormones and neurochemicals that alter body physiology and therefore human behavior. Odors are processed directly from the olfactory through the limbic system, a primitive part of the brain involved with the hypothalamus and having to do with emotions, memory, sexual behavior, and certain visceral activities. Therein lies the "pleasure center," the stimulation of which relates to primal behavior and the reinforcement of learning. Recent scientific evidence supports the observation that odors can help evoke memories, especially those with emotional overtones. Other senses also reach the limbic system but only after traveling to other regions of the brain.

The intriguing experimental olfaction research that has taken place internationally over the past decade, most particularly in the United States, has coincidentally paralleled the growth and rising interest in aromatherapy during the 1980s. Olfactory science has so far hearkened to the claims made for the psychological benefits of essential oils used in aromatherapy. A University of Cincinnati study showed that fragrances of peppermint and lily of the valley increased subjects' performance accuracy by 15 to 25 percent. A replication study at Catholic University using only peppermint achieved the same findings. It's becoming progressively clear that science and industry are convinced of the power of scent. But are they persuaded by aromatherapy? After-Flight Regulator essential oil blends, developed by aromatherapist Daniele Ryman to treat jet lag, are now offered at some London hotels and at the duty-free shop in Heathrow Airport's international terminal. Japanese construction firms are enhancing efficiency and reducing stress among office workers by pumping fragrances through air-conditioning systems. Junichi Yagi, a subsidiary vice-president for Shimizu, Japan's third largest construction firm, says that fragrances used by his company were selected by the principles of aromatherapy. In 1989, Dr. Gary Schwartz, current professor of psychiatry and psychology at the University of Arizona, found that spiced apple had relaxing effects, as measured in brain waves, within a minute of one subject's smelling that fragrance. It now is more critical for early researchers experimenting with many real and artificial scents, fragrances, and aromas to distinguish the mere stimulation of response from genuine therapeutic effects. Olfaction is so sensitive that virtually any odor will elicit brain response registering some clinically demonstrable physical or behavioral reaction, just as do electric stimuli; some may even prove beneficial. The crucial consideration is the relative value of those odors. Synthetic scents sometimes temporarily deceive the body, but as we have learned from the use of other artificial substances in food and medicine, the results are not genuinely positive and are not without negative consequences. If we acknowledge the folly of ingesting artificial ingredients and additives in our foods and the chemical synthetics of modern medicine, we ought to be no more eager to inhale inferior, synthetic, or artificial substances than we are to swallow them.

The profound and complete therapeutic effects of essential oils derive from more than their pleasant fragrance. They have vital electromagnetic properties and vibrational energies that invigorate the mind, the soul, the body's energy, and thus their functioning. When oils known for their sedative or antidepressant capacities are administered, endorphins and enkephalins (neurochemical analgesics and tranquilizers) are released. This has been demonstrated by hospitals in Oxford, England, where essential oils of lavender, marjoram, geranium, mandarin, and cardamom have replaced chemical sedatives. These and other oils relax people, lower blood pressure, increase mental acuity, normalize body functions, reduce stress, and even act as aphrodisiacs.

Serious olfaction research and experimentation involving essential oils will doubtless prove their superior efficacy. But if history is our guide, aromatherapists have reason to view with circumspection the olfaction research sponsored by fragrance companies, science labs, and medical institutions. Olfaction research is still in its infancy. We are only now gaining rudimentary appreciation of how and why essential oil fragrances affect human psychology and physiology even as we slowly trace the mysterious pathways of the brain. In this quest for knowledge, we would do well to adopt the reverential attitude of the early alchemists, for by olfaction research the psychology of scent may regain its vital spiritual and metaphysical heritage.

Thousands of scientists and researchers, as well as medical, beauty, and health professionals, working individually or as part of professional organizations, are already satisfied by aromatherapy, as are the millions of people, particularly in England, France, Germany, Belgium, and Switzerland, where aromatherapy is widely practiced. The United States, Canada, and Australia are the new frontiers. Another indication of aromatherapy's phenomenal rise over the past ten years is that as recently as fifteen years ago there were but one or two English-language aromatherapy books and few published articles. Today there are dozens and hundreds, respectively. All signs point to aromatherapy's ascendance to its rightful place as the premier health and beauty care system not just of this decade but of the next century.

# AROMATICS—FROM AROMATHERAPY TO PERFUMES

## A History Of Fragrance

During the past hundred years, the art of fragrancing practiced by modern perfumery, as we now define it, diverged from the original course of aromatics or from the holistic intentions and understanding now ascribed to modern aromatherapy. Ancient aromatherapy practiced before the discovery or general implementation of distillation—and therefore of pure essential oils—is more appropriately described as the practice of *aromatics:* the aesthetic or therapeutic use of scents or fragrances that are derived from plants but are not necessarily essential oils. Aromatics ought not be confused with modern perfumery involving fragrances that largely contain synthetic oils or scents diluted in alcohol and water, which merely smell pleasant or mask other odors. Unlike those of today, earlier advanced cultures and civilizations shared a more complex appreciation of fragrance, having a serious regard for the multiplicity of purposes, influences, and effects of aromatic substances. The straightforward intention of modern perfumery is to make people and things smell good or attractive.

19

Prehistoric or primitive man began using odoriferous materials to repel various predators, parasites, and natural invaders or to otherwise obscure or disguise himself and also to similarly offend or deceive his human enemies. He was far less likely to employ outside scents to identify himself or his tribe, let alone to inspire creativity or romance, preferring instead to rely upon his superior sense of smell (compared with that of modern, civilized man) to detect and discern natural human odors. As the increasing sophistication of human societies paralleled more complex human behavior and the advancement of knowledge, the use and perception of scent became less a concern for physical safety and survival and more a matter of socialization—i.e., of social acceptance, communication and conformity as well as social and personal identity. In addition, more advanced spiritual, aesthetic, psychological, and therapeutic purposes were eventually discovered for aromatic substances. Progressively more complex and developed human needs generated an increasingly more advanced understanding of aromatic substances and their vast capability to serve those needs. The evolving practice of aromatics began to uniquely display the amazing versatility and capacity of botanicals to satisfy the full spectrum of human physiological, psychological, aesthetic, social, and spiritual needs and motivations.

### Egypt

The ancient Egyptians were foremost in their extravagant use of fragrances. Like the Greeks, Romans, and later Europeans, the Egyptians designed personal perfumes to elicit various emotions and to inspire thoughts both in the wearer and in the intended admirer. Despite the crude distillation methods reportedly available in Egypt, these perfumes were customarily of unctuous (oily, fatty, or waxy) quality. Fragrancing was likewise used to honor, appease, and solicit favors from the gods; it was also linked to certain significant times and observances of the day, month, and year. In all instances, specific fragrances or scents were selected by special knowledge of correspondences. The appropriate selection of an aromatic oil or fragrance, whether to anoint a holy statue or an animal sacrifice, was made according to the deity being addressed and also the nature of the supplicant's entreaty.

Eventually, scents were created for nearly every purpose: to stimulate aggression during combat, to inspire spiritual ecstasy or deepen contemplation, to affix concentration and memory during study, and to arouse erotic sexuality, for example. It is said that Queen Hatshepsut (c. 1500 B.C), daughter of Thutmose I, was instrumental in advancing the use of cosmetics and perfumes among her subjects. The Egyptians also began to lace their beverages and liquids, such as beer, wine, and vinegar, with aromatics to increase their effects. More importantly, in Egypt as elsewhere in the Middle East and Asia, aromatics continued to expand socialization by substituting more intricate, adopted scents for natural human body odor. The pheromonal powers of human scent to communicate and attract had long been imperceptible owing to the decline of man's olfactory powers, but although the need for human scent had diminished, man's desire for fragrance had not.

### Greece and Rome

The ancient Greeks introduced the art of perfumery to the Romans, also transferring the traditional correspondences between certain kinds of fragrances and specific deities. The Greeks expanded the holistic reputation of aromatherapy by successfully applying aromatics to psychological conditions such as anxiety, depression, and hysteria as well as to artistic endeavors and other aesthetic pursuits of beauty and romance. Religious and spiritual exercises, such as meditation, prayer, consciousness expansion, and heightened perception and awareness were similarly improved by aromatics. The Greeks observed how incense and perfumes created conducive atmospheres for many spiritual, intellectual, creative, and romantic activities and experiences, intensifying their enjoyment. The thick smoke of incense, for example, lent itself to preserving thoughts and carrying spiritual messages and also to providing a medium for discarnate spirits—which kind depended on the type of incense or smoke. The tradition of ceremonial incense endures today in the Catholic Church and elsewhere. It's worth noting that in India the choice of sandalwood for temple construction was made not only because of sandalwood's material attributes and availability but because of its spiritual atmospheric affects as well.

It was generally understood by all societies utilizing aromatics that plants and their essences hold the key to purity and longevity. Still, the Greek democratic reformer Solon (c. 594 B.C.) actually restricted aromatics in the public places of Athens because he deemed their continual, indulgent use (and presumably their influence) too distracting. Centuries later, in Rome, Julius Caesar would feel compelled to do the same; although many years afterward, one of Caesar's more hedonistic successors, Emperor Claudius Nero, would lavishly surround and adorn himself and his palaces with roses.

Today, a new field of "environmental fragrancing" is emerging, not for the sake of beautification (or for medicinal purposes of fumigating cities against the spread of contagion, as the ancient Greeks and later the Europeans did) but as a kind of mass aromatherapy, to influence human psychological and social behavior collectively (e.g., to reduce theft or increase work performance). No doubt the social implications and propriety of this practice will invite the kind of scrutiny given to it in ancient Athens and Rome, but for now, discussion of environmental fragrancing must be postponed until we examine the psychology of scent.

### Europe
The European apothecaries were first to capitalize on the new botanical trade imports and knowledge of distillation brought home from the Middle East and North Africa by crusaders, merchants, and explorers during the period from the tenth to the fifteenth century. The new plant and essence imports fostered new interest in European perfumery, first noted in 1190 under the reign of the French king Philip II. Philip Augustus (as he was better known after his death in 1223) instituted guidelines for perfumery, requiring a four-year education in "essences" and subsequent performance testing before allowing anyone to practice the art.

The first major advance in modern aromatherapy and essential oil production began in the sixteenth century, when the specific use of distillation to obtain essential oils, not just floral waters, became prevalent. Consequently, all across Europe but especially in France, Italy, Germany, England, and Spain, the art of perfumery flourished, encouraged by European royalty. Catherine de Médicis, who served as royal regent of France from 1547 to 1589, set the fashion for perfumed gloves. Aromatic waters and potpourri became popularized under the auspices of Queen Elizabeth I of England, where special flower gardens were cultivated and floral sachets, usually sewn into ladies' skirts, became fashionable. Eventually, the entire nobility of Europe began using fragrances in a variety of ways, including oils, colognes, perfumes, pastes, powders, and pomades, to scent themselves as well as their clothing, jewelry, castles, and home furnishings.

Baths were quite popular among the Greeks and Romans. At one time, rose water actually ran via canals throughout Roman gardens and palaces. More than a thousand scented watering pools in the city accompanied unctuariums where bathers could be anointed and massaged with aromatic oils. Such hygienic customs did not readily spread to other European countries, such as England, where perfumery conveniently substituted for the unpopular practice of bathing. In Italy, where baths remained an honorable Roman tradition, the thriving soap industry was among the first to include the use of aromatics. The legendary French king Louis XIV ("le Roi Soleil"), whose reign from 1643 to 1715 was the longest in European history, was said to wear a new perfume each day. During his rule, the French perfume and soap industries began successfully competing with those from Italy. This development was perhaps encouraged by Louis himself, who at one time forbade perfumes altogether because their excessive use disguised the otherwise unsanitary habits of his people. It seems the French, like the English, too often neglected to bathe.

Meanwhile across the Channel, during the reign of Charles II, which began in 1660, a renowned perfumer named Charles Lily had written a book extolling the many virtues of fragrance. A century later, when George III ascended to the English throne, one of his first official acts was to ban perfumes in England, along with other cosmetic effects, because prostitutes were using them to seduce men. Indeed, it was judged that any woman attempting to seduce a man by means of "glamour" ought to be prosecuted for practicing sorcery. Such a peculiar edict was better appreciated in its day, when the supposedly nefarious practices of ritual magic and medieval alchemy had been known to include incense and perfumes.

### Modern Perfumery and Aromatherapy

The current interpretation of the word *perfume* illustrates the divergent course taken by modern fragrancing away from traditional aromatics and the present course maintained by modern aromatherapy. As recently as the nineteenth century, *to perfume* still meant "to disinfect"—to fumigate by using scent or, more literally, "through smoke" (per-fume). Both words, *fumigate* and *perfume*, derive from the Latin *fumus*, "smoke." Hence, the word *perfume* aptly describes something that floats like smoke. When ancient cultures and later European royalty scented themselves and their possessions, they did so not merely for adornment but also for their health. Floral or perfumed rooms, linens, and so on had not only psychologically uplifting benefits but germicidal and vermicidal effects as well. Even a casual floral bouquet ("nosegay") or scented handkerchief served this dual anti-infectious and mood-enhancing objective. Only in the past hundred years has the purpose of fragrancing, of perfumery, been divided between the somewhat aesthetic but largely cosmetic and commercial objectives of the modern perfume industry and the aromatically therapeutic objectives held by modern aromatherapy.

We know that the gradual rift between drug-oriented physicians and traditionally naturopathic, herbal physicians was inadvertently instigated in the mid-seventeenth century by enthusiastic alchemists who, by following the earlier lead of Paracelsus, saw marvelous possibilities for the chemicals discovered in their laboratories. The rift was widened by eighteenth-century and nineteenth-century chemists seeking to isolate chemical constituents (drugs) from plants, thus giving birth to the modern drug industry. Similarly, the late nineteenth-century and early twentieth-century chemists' exploration and analysis of the molecular structure and chemical components of essential oils spawned a new industry of isolated, synthetic aromatic substances—that is, modern perfumery. The important distinction is that no inherent competition or antagonism actually exists between modern perfumery and aromatherapy, save for perfumery's preposterous contentions about the comparative efficacy of synthetic versus natural essential oils. Indeed, modern aromatherapy owes much to the food and fragrance industries for the survival and progress of essential oil research. Conversely, modern perfumery owes its very existence to the 5,000-year tradition and development of aromatics and aromatherapy. Nonetheless, the peaceful coexistence of modern perfumery and aromatherapy relies less on their shared antecedents and more upon the fact that they serve different needs and ends.

### Steam Distillation and Alcoholic Perfumery

Modern perfumery and aromatherapy both owe their very existence to the development of steam distillation. First, by leading to the discovery and production of pure essential oils and of alcohol, steam distillation made possible the creation of non-oily perfumes. Also, it led to the inclusion of essential oils in alcoholic beverages, e.g., clary sage in German muscatel and Italian vermouth, and juniper in gin. Steam distillation, the process that medieval pharmacies used to produce floral waters (aromatic hydrosols) rather than essential oils, was a gradual development over a hundred-year period spanning the tenth and eleventh centuries. Principally motivated by the search for better aromatics, the use of distilled alcohol was largely directed toward expanding aromatherapy, besides creating alcoholic beverages. Alcoholic perfumery emerged from the mixture of alcohol and essential oils. Now, of course, modern perfumery includes synthetic or isolated aromatic chemical ingredients, but nonetheless it remains alcoholic perfumery. Today's commercial perfumes are composed of 15 to 20 percent concentrated "essence," the remaining 80 to 85 percent being alcohol and distillate water. For modern toilet waters the essence content is 6 percent, and for colognes it is approximately 3 to 5 percent, these products obviously containing proportionately larger percentages of alcohol and water. Perhaps needless to say, none of these manufactured fragrances is suitable for aromatherapy purposes.

### Perfume Ingredients

Initially, perfumers selected fragrance materials, extracted from animal sources, that are imitative of natural human secretions and thereby capable of simulating human sexual-olfactory signals: ambergris, a waxlike substance obtained from sperm whales; civet, a viscous yellowish secretion of the civet cat; and musk, a strong scent from certain male musk deer indigenous to Tibet, originally discovered by the ancient Chinese, who ascribed to musk healing powers. Later, myrrh, frankincense, and labdanum derived from plant sources were adopted, as were geranium, cypress, and then jasmine, tuberose, lilac, rose, and orange blossom (neroli), which are standards in classic French perfumery. Other perfumery favorites are lavender, bergamot, sandalwood, and amber. Because of their high cost, however, these natural fragrances have since been synthetically imitated by modern perfumers.

The aesthetic objective of traditional perfumery was to create harmony by balancing and blending ingredients. Today, the shift is toward a kind of symbiotic unification—active synthesis or dissonance, a scentual cohesiveness not necessarily at the expense of harmony, but not requiring it either. Dramatic rather than subtle effects are sought. This trend has generated a need and market for more synthetic components or chemicals that have exaggerated scents. The watchword in modern alcoholic perfumery is overdose, defined as an abundance of odoriferous energy.

## Perfume Formulation: Construction and Categories

The aromatherapist (or phytotherapist) creating an efficacious essential oil combination must take into account much more than its scent, and even at that the consideration of its therapeutic psychological, physiological, or spiritual affects outweighs the mere pleasantness of its collective fragrance.

The therapist must holistically evaluate the specific or multiple purpose of the essential oil selection, the administrative method of its application, and its exact use while selecting from the 100 to 150 essential oils the appropriate synergetic combination of 2 to 6 essential oils.

For the "nose" or commercial perfumer strictly designing an attractive, long-lasting fragrance, the choice of ingredients is made complex (even though the purpose and criteria are not) by the combined thousands of natural botanical essences, animal glandular extracts, and synthetic aromatic substances to choose from. Fortunately, the rules of perfume blending are fundamentally simple. While having to assess only the combined fragrance of ingredients, the nose selects and mixes scents much as a painter mixes colors. Regardless of the number of ingredients utilized in a given perfume, the construction pattern remains the same, resembling a basic three-note musical chord having a top or high note, a middle note, and a base or bottom note. Although referred to in the singular, each perfume "note" may include more than one, or even several, scent ingredients. In fact, some perfumes contain hundreds of ingredients.

### Perfume Construction

The *top note* requires light, highly evaporative, attention-getting ingredients, stimulating enough to create a brilliant first impression. The volatility of the top note, however distinctive, also guarantees that first scent impression will be short-lived, usually vanishing in five to ten minutes. The top note is vital to successful marketing of the perfume, particularly at the less expensive end of the perfume counter, where the top note is most relied upon to make the sale.

The less volatile *middle note* emerges after the top note fades. Also called the corps or core, the middle note is the heart of the perfume. To mimic a perfume's top note is easy, and it is often what competitors and cheaper copy perfumes do. But imitating the more subtle and complex middle note of a perfume requires identical ingredients in precise proportion.

The *base note* of a perfume comprises the heavy, more viscous, and slowly evaporative ingredients supplying a lingering scent. This is the deepest part of the complete fragrance. Base notes are fixative, but sometimes a fourth component is added to the basic three-note composition—another fixative or binder to further retard evaporation. (Then too, sometimes a fifth component, a neutral oil to dissolve or carry the other ingredients, is inserted into the mix. This is referred to as the diluent.) The total blend will determine how fast or slow the perfume fragrance unfolds to reveal itself. A good perfume usually lasts five or six hours. The endurance of toilet waters or colognes is proportionately less, owing to each's corresponding ingredient percentages of essence, alcohol, and water.

Clearly, the one similarity between a high-quality perfume formula and an aromatherapy essential oil combination is that each is not merely the sum of its parts but represents an active participatory relationship of those parts.

### Perfume Categories

One's evaluation of a scent is subjective, and the ability to express that evaluation is limited. The average person uses a scant few words to describe countless odors, scents, fragrances, and aromas. Even perfumers rely upon basic terms to identify or classify fragrances, which some say actually express just two fundamental qualities: seductive and sultry, or refreshing and stimulating. Nevertheless, those expressed qualities have several categories:

> *Single Floral*: a single flower scent, such as rose, jasmine, lilac, or gardenia, that is easy to wear and to identify.
>
> *Floral Bouquet:* a medley of light or heavy flower fragrances, none of which is foremost. Some of the most popular and familiar perfumes are floral bouquets; Joy and L'Air du Temps are two such florals.
>
> *Woodsy-Mossy:* sometimes referred to as herbal or "forest blend." A perfume from this category might contain sandalwood, rosewood, cedarwood, or balsam, perhaps combined with oak moss, fern, or other plants and herbs to attain an "outdoorsy" fragrance that is best appreciated on the wearer.
>
> *Fruity:* clean, refreshing fragrances based on fruit scents, such as peach, lime, lemon, or sometimes orange or apricot, usually blended in a citrus base.
>
> *Spicy:* pungent bouquets created from ingredients such as cinnamon, clove, ginger, and vanilla, and sometimes carnation.
>
> *Oriental:* sultry blends sometimes giving the impression of incense (for example, musk, civet, ambergris, or other exotic ingredients) and having deep, sophisticated tones that, depending on the

wearer, may be heady or somewhat overpowering. Shalimar and Opium are classic orientals.

*Modern Blend:* the newest trend toward liberally combining synthetic compounds and natural ingredients into unidentifiable scents; occasionally floral, woodsy, fruity, or spicy but characteristically having a stunning, indefinable, yet predominant top note. Many of the most costly and fashionably popular perfumes must be categorized as modern blends.

## The Objective Of Fragrancing

As upright man's sense of smell atrophied along with its declining significance to his individual experience and evolution (when compared with man's other senses), the civilized art of fragrancing generated stronger and stronger perfumes to substitute for natural human scent. Perfumery's mimicry of nature first began with erogenous scents maximizing physical attraction, and hopefully minimizing revulsion, to promote socialization—i.e., group identity, exclusivity, and procreation. Erotic perfumery evolved as the use of our sense of smell was diverted from serving the physical instinctive needs of basic survival toward satisfying our more complex emotional, social, and aesthetic motivations. This is now fully evident in the attempt of modern perfumery not to directly urge reproductive sex for the sake of the family or the species but instead to incite recreational sexuality with all its romantic allure and erotic fantasy. Perfumes are designed to exploit the passive, involuntary, and irrational (subconscious) sense of smell and to elicit emotional reactions via the limbic system (hypothalamus, amygdala)—the "old brain" governing primitive responses and hedonistic impulses of appetite, sexuality, and feelings. Although modern perfumery's specialized appeal to eroticism has no practical purpose, since we no longer instinctively smell for danger, we may as well smell for sensuous enjoyment, for pleasure, and for fun. Yet, there are other, more valuable and significant uses for our olfactory powers: opportunities to introspectively reveal, recreate, and savor memories and to expand imagination and creativity—superior, uniquely human traits that can be advanced by aromatherapy.

While moving from survival to socialization we have also moved from simplicity to saturation. By deliberate overdose we can now indulge our emotional and aesthetic responses to scents and fragrances, even while surrounded by odors and aromas exceeding our capacity to detect or accommodate, including our own. In a way, we have become artificially scented beings. To the extent that what we smell, and how we "smell," has slipped beneath our consciousness, we exaggerate and imitate olfactory stimuli to bring them into range of our perception. Ironically, although declining in acuity, our sense of smell has been advancing in sophistication, i.e., in the ability and desire to appreciate complex, intricate fragrances and aromas. What we have lost in olfactory intensity we have gained in aesthetic range. No longer rugged survivalists, we have become somewhat narcissistic olfactory dilettantes who regard smell more as a luxury than as a necessity.

Perfumers manipulate the thousands of natural and synthetic ingredients at their disposal in virtually limitless ways to gratify our personal and social tastes and also to escape mediocrity and sameness—to express themselves and ourselves. Perfumers are aware of how one perfume can smell differently on different people. Body chemistry is one reason; personal habits, diet, health, biological cycles, and environmental conditions are others. One's genetically programmed, physiological skin type is another determinant of satisfaction with a fragrance. Personal preferences may also mirror social preferences, e.g., a floral spice may be favored in France where lemon-lime is not, whereas in Germany the reverse is so. Although the many purposes, applications, methods, and uses of aromatics and perfumes have been remarkably alike from culture to culture and era to era, clearly different preferences for particular essences or fragrances remain. It would be incorrect to attribute those variations merely to chauvinism, geographic availability, or social habit and conditioning. Instead, they reflect genuine variety in human needs, desires, and inclinations, much as dietary or dress differences bespeak unique nutritional or climate requirements. Such differences and preferences, which may vary regionally or seasonally within the same society, are especially stark when homogeneous societies (e.g., Japan) are compared with pluralistic societies such as the United States. The perfume industry is both pleased and perplexed by the many marketing variables that determine the success or failure of a fragrance from one country, one region, one racial or ethnic group, or one person to the next. This is true not just for the cosmetic perfumers, who manufacture personal alcoholic fragrances, but also for the industry branch of functional perfumery, which since the 1950s has thrived by manufacturing scents conveying "cleanliness" and "freshness" and the like, first for inclusion in detergents, fabric softeners, and soap, and later other scents for everything else from candles to yarn. In fact, approximately 80 percent of modern perfume industry products are used to scent various items rather than people. Marketing long ago recognized how products that smell good, sell good.

## Popular Fragrances

It would be impracticable to completely and verifiably identify the quantity or quality of aromatic substances in the following recognizable name-brand and designer fragrances. Essence Rare (by Houbigant), for example, contains over 200 ingredients; Bal à Versailles more than three hundred. Countless commercial perfumes, toilet waters, and colognes have been produced in just this century. (Some sixty new perfumes are introduced each year by today's multi-billion dollar fragrance industry.) This list reveals some ingredients, natural and synthetic, of particular interest, perhaps providing some clues about your favorite fragrance.

| | |
|---|---|
| Ambush (Dana) | jasmine, rose, orchid, citrus |
| Arabesque (Merle Norman) | floral, musk, sandalwood, herb |
| A Rose Is a Rose Is a Rose (Houbigant) | Bulgarian rose otto, cognac |
| Bandit (Piguet/ Germaine Cellier) | wormwood |
| Belle de Jovan (Jovan) | orange blossom, rose, jasmine, carnation, violet |
| Blazer (Anne Klein) | hyacinth |
| Blue Grass (Elizabeth Arden) | jasmine, rose, violet |
| Bois des Iles (Chanel) | sandalwood |
| Boss Spirit (Hugo Boss) | wormwood |
| Chanel No. 19 (Chanel) | iris, jasmine, rose, ylang ylang, French moss, musk, sandalwood |
| Chantilly (Houbigant) | orange blossom, spice, chypre, sandalwood, vetiver, patchouli |

| | |
|---|---|
| Chloé (Karl Lagerfeld) | vetiver, oak moss, patchouli, jasmine, musk, tuberose |
| Diorella (Christian Dior) | vetiver, bergamot, honeysuckle, fern, patchouli |
| Essence Rare (Houbigant) | Bulgarian rose, patchouli, chamomile, fig leaf |
| Fidji (Lancome/ Guy Laroche) | rose, carnation, lilac, musk, jasmine, ylang ylang, ambergris |
| 4711 Eau de Cologne (Rorer Intl.) | lemon, lime, bergamot, tangerine, bitter orange blossom |
| Gentleman de Givenchy (Givenchy) | patchouli |
| Givenchy III (Givenchy) | amber, musk |
| Halston (Halston) | jasmine |
| Infini (Caron) | jonquil, lily, rose, jasmine |
| Interlude (Frances Denney) | rose, jasmine, patchouli, spice |
| Jontue (Revlon) | jasmine, tuberose, honeysuckle, jonquil |
| Joy (Patou) | rose absolute, jasmine absolute |
| L'Air du Temps (Nina Ricci) | carnation, Bulgarian rose, gardenia, jasmine |
| Le De (Givenchy) | jasmine, cyclamen, rose, fern, violet |
| Mackie (Bob Mackie) | jasmine, rose, jonquil |
| Madame Jovan (Jovan) | rose, jasmine, spice |
| Maja (Myrurgia) | rose, jasmine |
| Masumi (Coty) | mimosa, violet, rose, jasmine, geranium, hyacinth, muguet, sandalwood, vetiver, patchouli |
| Me (Vigny Parfums) | vetiver, sandalwood, musk |
| Monsieur Balmain (Germaine Cellier) | verbena |
| Muguet des Bois (Coty) | lily of the valley |
| My Sin (Lanvin) | orange blossom, patchouli |
| Nahema (Guerlain) | rose |
| 1,000 (Jean Patou) | violet |
| Orgia (Myrurgia) | rose, jasmine |

| | |
|---|---|
| Parure (Guerlain) | lilac, cypress, vetiver, plum |
| Realm (Germaine Monteil) | hyssop, ginger, balsam, clove, vetiver, olibanum, sandalwood, marjoram |
| Shalimar (Guerlain) | patchouli, vanilla, bergamot, iris |
| Society (Burberry) | orange blossom, tuberose |
| Tabu (Dana) | rose, jasmine, musk, amber |
| 20 Carats (Dana) | clove, rose, jasmine |
| V'E Versace (Gianni Versace) | ylang ylang, lily, Bulgarian rose |
| Vent Vert (Balmain/ Germaine Cellier) | galbanum |
| Vétiver de Guerlain (Guerlain) | vetiver |
| Via Lanvin (Lanvin) | jasmine, gardenia, narcissus, hyacinth |
| White Shoulders (Evyan) | violet, rose, tuberose, jasmine |
| Wind Song Breezy (Prince Matchabelli) | jasmine, rose, honeysuckle, spice, gardenia |
| "Y" (Yves St. Laurent) | ylang ylang |
| Yendi (Capucci) | musk, jasmine, honeysuckle, spice |

# 2

# Phytoaromatherapy and the Theory of Disease

## THE PHILOSOPHY OF HOLISTIC HEALING

The familiar holistic maxim "Treat the person, not the disease" expresses a fundamental philosophic and conceptual difference between conventional medicine (allopathy) and natural medicine (naturopathy). Allopathy is the study and treatment of disease; naturopathy is the study and treatment of health. In its war against disease, allopathy makes medicinal use of drugs, surgery, radiation, and other invasive (and seldom harmless) therapies. In seeking health, naturopathy embraces an enormously wide and diverse assemblage of natural, holistic therapeutics (e.g., diet and vitamin-mineral therapy, herbology, acupuncture, massage), including, of course, phytoaromatherapy. Holistic healing does not necessarily exclude allopathic methods but does consider them last-resort, crisis treatments rather than primary therapies. (In fact, medical officials themselves estimate that conventional medical intervention successfully aids patients only 10 to 12 percent of the time, and those results are almost entirely within the area of emergency/trauma medical care.) Hearkening to the Hippocratic injunction to "first, do no harm," naturopathy favors nontoxic and less hazardous remedies that present far less risk to the patient than do most conventional medical treatments. In this approach, holistic healing regards the person as a whole entity rather than as a collection of anatomical body parts. Hence, naturopathy treats the sick person, not the sick organ. This does not mean that holistic practitioners do not specialize, but they do so in their diverse approaches to the person or by their particular method of healing, not by specializing anatomically as do allopaths. Holistic healers cite each patient's personal responsibility for his or her own health, emphasizing preventive as well as corrective measures and the importance of lifestyle and attitudinal changes or adjustments necessary to the maintenance of good health—e.g., proper nutrition and exercise, correct elimination, clean fresh air, natural light, healthy psychological habits, and proper rest and relaxation.

Holistic healing differs from conventional allopathic medicine not only by its methodological treatment of illness but also by its perspective of disease itself. Long before technological etiology emerged in the late nineteenth century to assert the bacteriological origin of disease, the great naturopathic and holistic healers, while acknowledging the existence of bacteria and viruses, had rejected the notion that microorganisms are the primary cause of illness. Indeed, holistic healers, past and present, recognize no sole cause of illness but instead maintain that disease arises from a combination of factors involving disordered metabolism or organic malfunction.

Another basic tenet of holistic philosophy asserts that there is but one disease, regardless of what name it is given, that shows itself in various forms. A localized illness expresses a general state of ill-health, manifesting in whatever "weak link" may appear in one's chain of health depending upon one's predisposition. (By that we refer to normal genetic factors or natural predispositions, since most people are born healthy, rather than to congenital disease per se—the physical or metaphysical origins of which constitute another topic entirely that we cannot digress to explore.) When speaking of organic malfunction or disordered metabolism, we may more specifically infer that generalized disease results from autotoxemia (autointoxication) and enervation (deprivation or diminution of nerve force or energy), perhaps accompanied by preexisting or secondary nutritional and/or immunological deficiencies. "Illness is a process of degradation which precedes decomposition," says Dr. Valnet in *The Practice of Aromatherapy*. In the same book, Dr. Valnet quotes Rene Leriche: "Man brings about his illnesses by his own physiological means." To which we could add, by man's own psychological means too, since a great measure of disease and illness is psychosomatic; that is, it has strong psycho-physiological ties.

A localized disease, therefore, is a localized symptom requiring holistic, systemic therapy to truly remedy. This does not preclude localized "site-specific" corrective treatment. Holistic healing recognizes that particular tissues or organs subjected to long-term stress, neglect, or abuse may develop a chronic weakness or dysfunction that is not immediately amenable to generalized rehabilitative treatment but requires direct corrective care as well. Nevertheless, healing the whole person remains the primary objective, not merely stopping the symptomatic disease. As an holistic practice, phytoaromatherapy (the use of essential oils) offers both generalized (systemic) and localized (site-specific) remedies. Moreover, phytoaromatherapy is multilevel therapy, simultaneously acting upon the fourfold—physical, psychological (emotional and mental), and spiritual—human nature to achieve homeostasis (balance and harmony) within and among the four features.

## Homeostasis

Physiologically, homeostasis is the internal environment by which bodily states (e.g., blood circulation, biochemistry, respiration, digestion, temperature) are maintained at optimal levels for the survival and proper healthy functioning of a living organism. Based upon the principle of equilibrium that governs the body as a whole, homeostasis is autoregulatory, largely directed and maintained (biologically, at least) by the activities of the endocrine and autonomic nervous systems, but also involving numerous other metabolic systems and processes.

Homeostasis is, of course, responsive to stimuli such as fatigue, hunger, thirst, and a variety of external or internal factors and agents. Homeostasis can be disturbed by poor or wrong diet; by physical or emotional stress, exertion, or upset; and by toxication from medicines, environmental pollutants, or other toxic external agents. Drugs, despite the best corrective intentions, greatly disturb and impair homeostasis, as do emotional behavioral extremes. Conversely, by their hormonal, innervative (electromagnetic/etheric), nutritive, and other therapeutic properties and capabilities, essential oils help restore, normalize, and maintain homeostasis.

# EXPERIMENT AND EXPERIENCE WITH ESSENTIAL OILS

These two approaches—experiment and experience—toward gaining knowledge about essential oils are neither mutually exclusive nor dependent; they are independent yet cooperatively valuable methods of essential oil research. But, in the end, after each is given the opportunity to explore the nature and efficacy of essential oils, experiment (lab testing and analysis) must give way to experience or empirical evidence. Empirical evidence must be the final determinant about whether or not something "works," irrespective of whether experiment is capable of showing how or why it works. The common modern assumption that lab experimentation can infallibly prove or demonstrate the worth and workings of everything is itself erroneous. Fortunately, phytoaromatherapy's efficacy does not rely altogether upon experimental verification or evidence. It is instructive to remember that not all things useful or beneficial can be tested or demonstrated in the experimental lab. Conversely, many things proved experimentally effective within the limited measure and expectations of the lab are not necessarily useful or beneficial; something that works in the lab, *in vitro*, may not work (or work safely) in real-life application, *in vivo*. For one thing, substances or chemicals do not behave in the body as they behave in the lab.

In these modern times too, one is likewise conditioned to routinely expect lab experimentation to test and validate experience or empirical evidence, when in fact the reverse is inevitably required. Regardless of the supposed merits of the recipe, the proof of the pudding is in the tasting. Still, the value of lab analysis and experimental research, especially of testing new, untried substances about which little or no experiential or empirical evidence exists, ought not be underestimated. Science improves itself each day, expanding its range of perception, which admittedly has a long way to go considering the range of possibilities in this world, let alone the universe.

How laboratory science applies itself to the understanding of essential oils is of great importance to phytoaromatherapy. By its own limitations or inadequacies—whether analytical, attitudinal, methodological or procedural—and by failing to see the forest for the trees, lab science could wrongly assess an essential oil as "unsafe" or "ineffective" when in fact, by empirical evidence, it is neither. This sometimes happens when isolated

36

chemical constituents of an essential oil are tested rather than the naturally complete essential oil as it would actually be administered. Consider too that toxicology tests on animals or on isolated human tissue are often misleading. First, animals are not human. Animals and humans metabolize differently, hence what may prove toxic for laboratory mice may not be so for humans. Second, internal organ tissue would never in actuality be exposed to substances in such a way. Internal tissue lacks the protective metabolic "screening" capacity of skin tissue, which is discriminatory and transformational. Ironically, by such testing methods, harmless, beneficial substances (not just essential oils) have been unjustly condemned or dismissed as hazardous or ineffective, while numerous drugs deemed experimentally safe later reveal themselves to be extremely dangerous and/or utterly useless. All too often such drugs remain on the market because they are otherwise profitable. It is common enough that theoretically or experimentally devised medical remedies or procedures (drugs, radiation, chemotherapy, or experimental surgery) prove ineffective or harmful in actual practice, yet the use of those medicines and procedures is allowed to continue despite the experientially or empirically known risks and demonstrable side-effects. The perpetuation of bad medicine is as much motivated by profit and power as it is an unfortunate, unintended consequence of poor scientific judgement. If scientific empiricism were equally applied in all cases, many profitable but harmful and/or useless conventional medical therapies would disappear tomorrow from the medical marketplace, pharmacies, and hospitals.

## Pharmacology and Essential Oils

The currently fashionable use of the term *pharmacological* to describe the psycho-physiological activity of essential oils is perilously misleading and inappropriate. While seeming to lend sophistication and legitimacy to essential oil applications and effects, the term demeans the spirit of phytoaromatherapy and plays carelessly into the hands of those whose untrustworthy motives are incongruous with the holistic inclinations and therapeutic activities of naturopathy. The naturally biochemical, physiological, or psychological activity of a natural organic substance, such as a food, an herb, or an essential oil, cannot and ought not be described as "pharmacological," literally meaning "to act as a drug." Pharmaceutical drugs have pharmacological action. Essential oils are not pharmaceuticals. The use of this term reveals the kind of mechanistic thinking that led to drug therapy in the first place, similar to thinking that the eye operates like a camera or that the body works like a machine. By such comparisons we ought to wisely consider which came first, then conclude that such thinking is backward. Mention of their "pharmacological" activity makes it sound as if essential oils are imitating drugs, when it is quite the reverse: drugs "work" because they mimic or usurp the activity or role of natural substances such as essential oils. But drugs have false and unnatural effects. The effects of essential oils are naturally bioactive, biotic, psychoactive, and psychotherapeutic; but they are definitely not "pharmacological," which is the wrong yardstick and wrong terminology to descriptively compare the marvelously complex operation of an essential oil to the heavy-handed, one-dimensional effects of a drug. Certainly, after complete consideration of all the pharmacological effects attributable to drugs, we should be further pleased and thankful that essential oils have no such "pharmacological" activity.

The normalizing activity (homeostatic intelligence) of essential oils does not submit to the limited pharmacological view that sees a single-action drug having a single effect. Unlike drugs, essential oils respect and intelligently communicate with living tissue. Seemingly contradictorily, an essential oil will stimulate a hypoactive organ or stabilize one that is hyperactive, restoring homeostasis. Angelica, for example, either relaxes or contracts the uterus, depending on the condition or need. Drugs unintelligently disrupt homeostasis, causing collateral damage or side-effects along with harm by their single-action intents. Other essential oils having normalizing (balancing and stabilizing) effects in various psycho-physiological processes, systems, and conditions, (e.g., hormonal, emotional, blood pressure, skin) include geranium, niaouli, vetiver, bergamot, fennel, jasmine, neroli, black spruce, garlic, and hyssop. By their nature, properties, and effects, essential oils are too complex, too multidimensional, too versatile, and too intelligent to be pharmacologically pigeonholed by medical science.

## Essential Oil Safety

Competitors of phytoaromatherapy, having their own jealous, monopolistic agenda for human health care, would like to see essential oils severely restricted if not banned outright. To accomplish this, they eagerly promote irrational doubts and fears about essential oils, ostensibly in the interest of public safety. Even among practitioners there are the pretentious few whose exaggerated claims about the "hazardous" and "pharmacological" nature or effects of essential oils are intended to impress us with the seriousness of their knowledge and serve their authoritative ambitions in the field, but do little to serve phytoaromatherapy or the public. Meanwhile, the more conscientious therapists, who have responsible, reasonable concerns about comparatively few and seldom-used essential oils, continue to advance the success of phytoaromatherapy. Several highly active, but safe essential oils have already been tagged as scapegoats or sacrifical lambs by the alarmist factions. We are reminded of the recent basil controversy and of how the incomplete analysis of sage's chemical constituents prompted unwarrantable concerns about its toxicity. Thyme has also been a victim of dubious toxicity research. Juniper is occasionally maligned by false rumors of toxicity and abortifacience owing to a simple case of mistaken identity that apparently originated in 1928, when because of a similarity of Latin names, juniper (*Juniperus communis*) was mistaken for savin (*Juniperus sabina*). They are not the same plant or oil, nor are they chemically similar. Other oils have likewise been misrepresented, been misanalyzed, or had demonstrable empirical evidence of their safety ignored. Some essential oils are rightfully excluded from aromatherapy (if not from phytotherapy) as unsuitable for inhalation or topical use, but even they have medicinal or phytotherapeutic value and are otherwise safe when used wisely and moderately by informed practitioners.

## OBSTETRIC AROMATHERAPY

After reading repeated warnings, one might think that no essential oil should ever be used during pregnancy. Not only is such an assumption erroneous, but there are many safe essential oils that correctly applied, especially by inhalation or massage, are uniquely beneficial for obstetric purposes. For countless generations, herbs and essential oils have been extensively employed during pregnancy, parturition, and postnatal care to relieve pain, to stimulate uterine contractions (labor), to improve the health of the mother and child by enhancing immunity or by protecting both against toxic elements and infection, to ensure healthy fetal development, to stem excessive bleeding, to promote lactation, and to alleviate psychological conditions. Ironically, while today's public and professional ignorance of traditional herbs and essential oils invites much suspicious caution about their use, many pregnant women continue to indiscriminately partake or indulge in all sorts of potentially harmful activities, practices, or substances—tobacco, alcohol, prescription and nonprescription drugs, polluted or toxic exposure, excessive hot tub use, bad nutrition—often without caution from their physicians.

Fortunately, the wonderful benefits of aromatherapy for women are well chronicled in the writings of several authors—Maggie Tisserand, Valerie Ann Worwood, and Patricia Davis among them—who provide valuable information about obstetric and pediatric aromatherapy care. Essential oil remedies and formulas for morning sickness, psychological depression or anxiety, stretch marks, fainting, cramps, circulatory complaints and edema, and virtually every other condition of pregnancy or childbirth are thereby available. The resurgence of natural birth and home birth techniques and midwifery has been instrumental in the reemergence of herbs and essential oils in obstetrics. This is especially true in Europe, where obstetric and pediatric aromatherapy is better appreciated.

## Prenatal Toxicology

The study of the prenatal toxicity of foreign substances, particularly drugs, remains inexact because of the uniqueness of the human reproductive system and the complexity of human biology in comparison with other animals or mammals used for test studies, and also because human experiments are too risky and virtually impossible to conduct, which is why animals are used in the first place. It is therefore difficult to predict, especially by animal experimentation, which substances will reach the developing child in the womb via the mother's blood circulation or what the effects may be.

In the case of essential oils it has been presumed that toxicity and emmenagogic activity usually combine to classify an essential oil as abortifacient, and not merely its emmenagogic activity alone. (Savin oil, for example, has produced uterine stimulation indicating its emmenagogic, hence abortifacient, potential, but it is savin's toxicity that is as much or more a health concern.) Yet, those oils thereby classified have shown marked unreliability as abortifacients; even when they work sporadically, it now seems evident that so-called "abortifacient" essential oils are effectively so only when ingested in toxic dosages. Substance toxicity, most typically by ingestion, is very much dosage dependent.

Having antiseptic, carminative, sudorific, emmenagogic, analgesic, febrifugal, and expectorant properties, and capable of treating numerous ailments, pennyroyal has been an effective medicinal herb for at least 2,000 years. Today, pennyroyal's reputation is principally as a notorious abortifacient. Yet, there is no real documented empirical evidence that one can cause an abortion with pennyroyal short of ingesting a lethal or very nearly lethal dose, which in the case of its essential oil would certainly be within one ounce. This means that by using pennyroyal to accomplish an abortion, a woman would be deliberately or unintentionally committing suicide, since abortion will consequently occur from deadly poisoning, just as it would from any other toxic substance. Indeed, were a woman willing to risk suicide from deadly poisoning in an attempted abortion, she could more readily do so by ingesting any one of the numerous substances available on supermarket or pharmacy shelves, rather than by swallowing oil of pennyroyal. Nevertheless, despite its great therapeutic value, pennyroyal's potential toxicity, not its reputed abortifacience, categorizes it as a hazardous oil.

## Hazardous Essential Oils

These listed essential oils are easily avoided, since they have little or no applicative use in aromatherapy. Their oral toxicity (rather than simple topical irritation or sensitization), hence sometimes more specifically their potential as convulsants or abortifacients, generally precludes their use at any time but especially during pregnancy or other obstetrical (OB) processes and procedures. Otherwise, they ought not be administered except under expert supervision.

> Boldo: toxic
> Calamus: toxic (convulsant)
> Horseradish: toxic
> Hyssop: toxic (convulsant)
> Mugwort: toxic (abortifacient)
> Mustard: toxic
> Pennyroyal: toxic (OB toxic)
> Rue: toxic (abortifacient, convulsant, OB toxic)
> Savin: toxic (abortifacient, OB toxic)
> Tansy: toxic (OB toxic)

Thuja: toxic (abortifacient, convulsant)
Wintergreen: toxic (convulsant)
Wormseed: toxic (convulsant)
Wormwood: toxic (convulsant)

Other oils are occasionally suspected of lesser toxicity, but the experimental evidence is inconclusive, and experience has shown little cause for concern. Although generally safe, certain distinctly hormonal, more specifically estrogenic oils or those that affect lactation (e.g., hops, licorice, cypress, angelica, fennel, anise seed, sage, lemongrass, and coriander) and similarly nontoxic but emmenagogic oils should most probably be avoided during pregnancy.

## THE TOPICAL USE OF ESSENTIAL OILS

As Dr. Valnet reminds us in *The Practice of Aromatherapy*, "The skin's absorptiveness has always been exploited in the treatment of general conditions (e.g., with iodine paint or friction rubbing with liniments based on garlic, olive oil, or camphor)." Naturally lipid-soluble substances, essential oils are highly skin permeable, but many other factors can determine the rate and efficacy of essential oil absorption.

### Transdermal Factors

Skin permeability varies according to body area and greatly involves the relative efficiency and thoroughness of blood (capillary) circulation. The hands, feet, scalp, forehead, and armpits or underarms are most permeable. Generally, those body areas providing easiest skin access are those with more hair follicles and sweat glands or that have high blood circulation. We are reminded that massage, by increasing circulation, also increases essential oil absorption. The viscosity of the massage carrier oil is another determinant of absorption. A good carrier oil dilutes and diminishes the volatility of essential oils thereby adjusting their absorption rate. Conversely, the carrier oil's own skin saturation also sustains that absorption. Like warm hands or a warm ambient temperature, a warm oil furthers essential oil absorption. But since heat increases evaporation and the likelihood of damage to the essential oil, and to the carrier, it is best not to apply artificial warmth to the oils. When room-temperature oils are used, the naturally generated warmth from the hands and friction will suitably vaporize the essential oils, providing through inhalation other benefits from the aromatic massage. Dry, open pores, after a bath or steam will increase absorption. Of course, actual sweating decreases absorption by its diluting and washing effects.

Diseased epidermal tissue usually permits greater absorption than does healthy skin. Abnormal (rapid or slow) skin permeability may also be induced by drugs administered by ingestion or otherwise. Finally, draping the skin with a covering after localized treatment will enhance absorption by reducing the evaporation of volatile substances such as essential oils.

The skin, the largest organ of the body, is a highly selective, discriminatory metabolic organ. It is neither a sieve nor a stone wall. It possesses its own peculiar enzymes that transform topically applied substances, either detoxifying them or somehow chemically altering them either for access or elimination. Naturally salutary substances, such as essential oils, are made readily accessible to the body by the skin. Whereas topical dermal irritation or sensitization is possible from some essential oils, transdermal toxicity akin to oral toxicity is virtually nonexistent. When one is selecting an essential oil for topical application, not only should its inherent therapeutic value and possible contraindications be considered but also its dosage (amount, dilution, and frequency of use) as well as other factors such as gender differences. Women are more thin-skinned than men. Their skin being more permeable, women are more susceptible to transdermal passage of toxic chemicals and other foreign substances. Moreover, male perspiration is more acidic than that of women, and is therefore naturally more bactericidal and more capable of disrupting or neutralizing noxious substances. Also, by natural requirement, women have twice the percentage of body fat, averaging 20 to 25 percent, compared with 10 to 15 percent for men. Such facts have important implications for the relative effectiveness of aromatherapy massage and topical essential oil therapy as well as for the relative toxic resistance of men and women in other circumstances.

In his book *Principles of Holistic Therapy with Herbal Essences*, Dr. Dietrich Gümbel introduces his own adaptation of the law of correspondences or principle of similarity. Basing his skin therapy on a physiological comparison between plants and man, specifically correlating the metabolism of plant flowers, sprouts, and roots to the three layers (epidermal, dermal, and subcutaneous) of human skin, Dr. Gümbel also notes a continued correlation among upper, middle, and lower plant parts, the layers of human skin, and the three divisions of the human body—head, upper body, and lower body. Dr. Gümbel's simple theory and system of applying essential oils derived from a specific part of the plant (flowers, fruit, leaves, bark, roots) to benefit a corresponding layer of the skin or sectional area of the body offers a somewhat unusual method of essential oil selection (although there are other variations of this idea in phytotherapy). We do not necessarily recommend his method but do think it is worth mentioning for the insight it provides.

To practice safe, accurate, and efficient phytoaromatherapy, one must make the correct selection of essential oils by first learning all that can be known about the oils themselves, including, of course, each oil's own properties and nature, then, too, its botanical identity, its source, the method and duration of extraction, and how it has been otherwise prepared, preserved, or handled. Good quality essential oils are important to the correct practice of phytoaromatherapy, as is the proper dosage and method of application for correctly selected oils. There is also the matter of therapeutic purpose, which most importantly involves the person and illness to be treated. In phytoaromatherapy, as in other naturopathic practices, the right treatment (essential oil selection, dosage, method of application) is ultimately determined by knowing the person and knowing the etiology, implications, and extent of the illness by its systemic and/or localized nature and features.

## CLINICAL PHYTOAROMATHERAPY

Ever since the action of terebinth (turpentine) against the anthrax bacillus was first observed by Koch in 1881, and subsequent French studies of other essential oils were commenced by Chamberland, Cadeac and Meunier, and Bertrand in 1887, hundreds of lab tests have reaffirmed the antiseptic and microbicidal (antimicrobial) properties of essential oils. Every essential oil has such properties, but some are more or less effective against a specific bacterium than are others. Too, some essential oils have a wider spectrum of antimicrobial efficacy. One such oil is tea tree, which is deadly not only to streptococci, gonococci, and pneumococci, but to the *Candida albicans* fungus and the single-cell *Trichomonas vaginalis* parasite. Moreover, tea tree, like other essential oils, is antiviral.

44

The wide-ranging microbicidal effects of various essential oils, as demonstrated by successful test results, include cinnamon against the typhus bacillus, clove bud against *Mycobacterium tuberculosis*; sandalwood and lemongrass against *Staphylococcus aureus*, and lemon oil against meningococcus, staphylococcus, streptococcus, and pneumococcus germs, typhus bacillus, and *Corynebacterium diphtheriae*. German chamomile has proved effective against *Staphylococcus aureus, Proteus vulgaris,* and hemolytic streptococcal infections. Another excellent antiseptic, thyme oil, is effective against *Escherichia coli,* the typhus bacillus, and streptococcus, diphtheric, staphylococcus, and tuberculosis germs. The amazing versatility of so many essential oils has led French physicians to develop and rely upon a new lab test method of targeting specific microbes with essential oils.

## The Aromatogram

The aromatogram is a lab test that allows phytotherapists to analyze *in vitro* the antibacterial activity of essential oils and to more accurately select those essential oils best able to suppress or destroy the targeted germs. This test method is conducted much like the conventional culture test (antibiogram) used by allopathic physicians to observe the effects of antibiotics. For those unfamiliar with the antibiogram, Dr. Valnet, in *The Practice of Aromatherapy*, describes the procedure:

> It consists of bringing together on selected culture media in a laboratory the offending infectious agents and a number of different substances (both chemical and natural) in order to ascertain the degree of effectiveness of the different products on the germs in question.

As history and Dr. Valnet remind us, the suppression of germs *in vitro* by essential oils was not discovered yesterday, and the gradual development of the aromatogram has many contributors. Perhaps the most notable among them, Dr. Maurice Girault, a French gynecologist and obstetrician, published the result of his six years of test research involving essential oils and plant tinctures by which he first demonstrated clinical phytotherapy's own version of the antibiogram.

First, Dr. Girault gathered vaginal secretions on a swab to identify the offending microbes and placed them in cultures, later introducing different essential oils to determine which of them proved most effective against the identified microorganisms. A more detailed account of the aromatogram is offered by Dr. Valnet in his aforementioned book:

> The process involves testing various aromatic oils on germs iso-lated by the culture method, from a liquid or piece of organic mate-rial taken from a sick person. To do this, you pour some agar into a Petri dish and place on it some discs impregnated with oils.
>
> Then you sub-culture the germ in the usual media for 24 hours—long enough for the culture to develop and fill the Petri dish—which is what actually happens, except in the areas occupied by the oils which have an inhibitive action on the germ. The scale runs from 0 to 3 ac-cording to the diameter of the area affected by the inhibitors [the *zone of inhibition*]* and the result is expressed, as in the case of the antibi-ogram, according to the degree of sensitivity of the germ to the oil.

The aromatogram method first employed by Dr. Girault has since been further applied to all types of infection from which cultures can be gath-ered. The valuable microbicidal, antiseptic properties of essential oils, pre-viously demonstrated for nearly a century, now can be specifically microbe-targeted, making essential oils more effective still. In each case, infectious material is taken on a swab from a patient's infected location and cultured in the lab. The bacteria are allowed to multiply, and then as many as a dozen essential oils are tested before the choice of oils to be given is nar-rowed down. The patient is treated either by ingestion (orally), by inhala-tion (transpulmonary), or topically (transdermally/percutaneous), the two other clinical phytoaromatherapy methods being injection and supposi-tory insertion. In the presence of more than one microbe, when it is un-known exactly which bacterium is solely or chiefly responsible for the in-fection, the selected essential oil combination of 2 to 6 oils will span the remedial requirement.

---

*The *zone of inhibition* describes the circle around each of the essential oils placed on the culture in the clear Petri dish. The diameter of the circle (measured in millimeters) show-ing the bactericidal area of the oil determines the oil's efficacy. The larger the diameter, the greater the bactericidal effect. No circle, no effect.

## Limitations of the Aromatogram

Perhaps needless to say, the aromatogram has greatly expanded clinical phytotherapy's treatment of infectious and allergic diseases. But, as Dr. Jean-Claude Lapraz cautions, it is, after all, just another lab test providing the clinician with complementary information; it does not by itself constitute or represent a diagnosis, least of all a diagnosis of the patient. Simply stated, the purpose of the aromatogram is to ascertain *in vitro* which essential oils are to be considered for treatment of the patient, a selection procedure that actually begins with the informed and knowledgeable choice of essential oils to be tested in the first place. The choice of essential oils is substantially improved by consideration of various criteria gathered from the aromatogram and from other sources. All other characteristics of an essential oil, not just its antimicrobial properties, are considered. Always, attention is given to the site, etiology, and prognosis of the illness or disease; more importantly, the actual condition of the patient is studied. The aromatogram brings together the opportunistic microbe(s) and selected essential oil to provide an indication of the essential oil's bactericidal capability against the offending germs in question. But there is a third all-important factor in the health and treatment equation about which the aromatogram tells us nothing: the host, which is the patient, or clinically speaking, the *terrain*. By Dr. Lapraz's definition, "Terrain is the potential makeup of the genetic elements which have modeled the organism in a certain structured neuro-endocrinal state, and a particular functional structure which is the result of these genetic elements." Others, such as Drs. Valnet and Penoel, might explain the concept of terrain somewhat differently, but the term *terrain* describes the inherently unique psycho-physiological disposition, makeup, and current status of the patient and consequently too of the patient's cells, tissues, organs, and systems.

Logically, the host, or patient, must be analyzed in ways other than by the aromatogram. The patient ought to be holistically examined by conventional or unconventional means and methods that evaluate the patient's general systemic health and condition (homeostatic state) as well as the localized, symptomatic manifestation of illness. The devised treatment of designated essential oils is then applied locally, regionally, and/or systemically by whichever of the five phytoaromatherapeutic methods is considered appropriate.

47

It must be remembered that owing to its complex qualities and other properties, an essential oil's observable effects upon a germ *in vitro* are not exactly the same as those upon or within the patient, which is why the entire nature of the essential oil, to whatever extent it is known, must be evaluated for correct selection and not just the information gathered from the aromatogram. The behavior of an essential oil can be anticipated *in vitro* but must be further observed *in vivo*, owing not only to the complexity of the oil but to the variance of the terrain. Moreover, as Dr. Valnet indicates in his book, "a well-known and neatly classified microbe is not necessarily identical to its homologue harbored by a different host. For instance, the coli bacillus present in one patient may respond to the essential oil of pine and in another patient to lavender or thyme." These behavioral peculiarities highlight the significance of the terrain and the indispensability of individualized treatment. There is no substitute for personal knowledge of the patient . . . or of the essential oils.

## SPECIAL FACTORS AND VALUES: PH, $RH_2$, RESISTANCE

The infected swab's pH (potential hydrogen) value is also calculated in the aromatogram, its degree of acidity or alkalinity revealing information about the microbe and the milieu of the infection. Measured on a scale between 0 to 14, the pH value represents the relative acidity or alkalinity of a solution or substance. The lower the pH number, the greater the acidity of the solution. Pure distilled water (HOH) is virtually neutral (pH 7.0); clean rain water is naturally acidic, ranging between pH 5.0 and pH 5.5.

All the body's chemical processes depend upon homeostatic maintenance of a delicate pH balance between hydrogen (H) and hydroxyl (OH) ions in the blood. Hydrogen (H) is acid-forming, and oxygen (O) forms alkali; hydrogen combined with oxygen in a hydroxyl group (OH) creates an alkaline reaction. Too many hydrogen ions create acidosis; too few will cause alkalosis. Water (HOH) is neutral, but the optimal pH figure for human blood is a slightly alkaline 7.4. Actually, healthy human blood narrowly fluctuates between pH 7.38 and pH 7.42, delicately controlled by the homeostatic system regulating acidity through respiration (and other organs and systems, e.g., the kidneys). Too much acidity increases respiration to discharge carbon dioxide ($CO_2$) and increase oxygen; too much alkalinity decreases respiration to retain $CO_2$ and increase hydrogen ions in the blood. It is noteworthy that hydrogen thickens solutions, whereas oxygen thins them. This is obviously relevant to the ease and efficiency of cardiovascular blood circulation and to other systems and processes, such as digestion. Since hydrogen causes substances to clump or stick together, whereas oxygen thins or separates them so they can be assimilated, hydrogenated foods, especially hydrogenated fats, are thicker and harder on the system. By their particular nature, foods create acid or alkaline reactions in the body. For example, meats, fish, peanuts, and cranberries are acid-producing; most fruits and vegetables are alkaline-producing. Some foods are neutral. Proper food combining is a somewhat involved nutritional science, but generally speaking, the best foods are those having the most or highest percentage of oxygen: in descending order, complex carbohydrates (more than 50 percent), proteins (20 to 50 percent), fats (10 to 15 percent). "Fat acidosis" is common because fats not only are oxygen deficient but are oxygen robbers. Drugs also rob oxygen.

The pH scale is logarithmic, like the Richter earthquake scale: the difference from one number on the scale to the next (2 to 3, for example) represents a tenfold difference in hydrogen ion concentration. A two-number difference (2 to 4) represents a hundredfold difference. The disinfectant qualities of lemon juice and vinegar are partly attributable to their similar acidic pH values, which approach that of stomach acid. Correct stomach acid pH ranges from 1 to 3 (1.8 to 2.3). A pH 1.0 solution (e.g., hydrochloric acid) will destroy most bacteria and seriously disrupt the molecular structure of numerous noxious substances.

The $rH_2$ factor defines the electron charge of a given pH value (for which there can be an infinite number of $rH_2$ values) and the power of oxido-reduction (antioxidance), which is the variant balance between oxidation and reduction in the body—the balance of oxygen and hydrogen. The $rH_2$ scale is 0 to 42, the value differences being quite narrow. *Resistance* is the capacity of a solution or substance to oppose the transmission of electricity. The resistance scale is quite wide; for example, essential oils have values measured in the thousands, whereas human blood resistance is expressed in hundreds.

Essential oils have a decidedly acid pH, another feature of their bactericidal activity. Acidity opposes microbial multiplication or proliferation; alkalinity encourages it. Essential oils also have a high resistance, which discourages the spread or diffusion of infections and toxins. The $rH_2$ factor of an essential oil varies according to the oil, which may activate oxidation or reduce it appropriately. Thus, an essential oil can be antimicrobial and powerfully oxidizing (e.g., peppermint) or antioxidant while antiviral and anticarcinogenic (e.g., clove).

Experimental studies of essential oils, beginning with those having a culinary reputation (e.g., clove, garlic, thyme, nutmeg, pepper) reveal their anti-aging effects conferred by their antioxidant capabilities, which protect tissues from the ravages of oxidant free radicals. An oxidant free radical is a renegade or delinquent atom, or cluster of atoms (molecule), with an unpaired or odd electron that damages healthy cells through lipid peroxidation (improper combustion, assimilation of fats) or other free radical production by exposure to radiation, pollutants, or chemical substances (e.g., drugs) or originating from emotional or physical stress. Free radical oxidation is associated with cytotoxicity, disease, and aging in human beings. It is instructive that free radicals are not produced from too much oxygen but are actually the offspring of inadequate and/or incomplete oxygenation caused by toxic intrusions, nutritional deficiency, or poor metabolic functioning—in short, from too many toxins and too little oxygen to accomplish metabolic, physiologic tasks. The body's response to oxidant free radicals is to produce antioxidant enzymes or to seek natural substances and foods with antioxidant enzyme/coenzyme properties.

Essential oil mixtures seem to compound their innate acidity, collectively lowering their pH, and to magnify resistance—another demonstration of the marvelous synergystic activity of essential oil blends. Dr. Valnet gives much credence to the significance of the high resistance of essential oils. Professor Paolo Rovesti likewise notes that the electromagnetic molecular charge of essential oils has "a sharp influence on cellular magnetic fields." Clearly, the implications of their pH, $rH_2$, and resistance offer another insight into the therapeutic effects of essential oils. As Rovesti notes, the presence of cancer accompanies a reduced electrical resistance in cells. Cancer is also linked to excessive free radical damage (of oxidation) caused by excess toxification and cellular oxygen deficiency or asphyxiation. Apparently, then, the anticarcinogenic properties of clove oil, for example, have much to do with clove's very high resistance (4,000), low $rH_2$ value (16.5) and acidic pH (6.7).

# GARLIC (*ALLIUM SATIVUM*)

Certainly one of the most famous and researched remedies ever, garlic has for centuries been widely employed as an antibacterial, antifungal, and antiviral agent against virtually every contagious and infectious disease in history, including tuberculosis, diphtheria, and the plague. The list of microorganisms sensitive to garlic is too long to recite. A truly wonderful and completely safe herb, garlic is also a vermifuge against intestinal worms and parasites.

The clinically demonstrated power of garlic oil (oleum alii) to inhibit early cell changes associated with colon cancer, as well as benign and malignant tumor growth there and elsewhere in the body has been widely reported during the past several years. By possessing both antioxidant and pro-oxidant (oxygenation) capabilities, garlic evinces the seemingly contradictory characteristics of homeostatic intelligence typical of essential oils. As an immune stimulant or regulator, garlic is also helpful for autoimmune diseases, such as systemic lupus erythematosus (SLE). The normalizing powers of garlic extend further to its effect upon blood pressure (hypotension or hypertension) and other cardiovascular activities. Garlic is indicated for artherosclerosis and lipidemia (elevated cholesterol and triglyceride levels); it also inhibits abnormal blood platelet aggregation (clotting). Garlic's blood-thinning properties are also attributable to its dissolving effect upon uric acid.

# THERAPEUTIC EFFECTS OF ESSENTIAL OILS

Dr. Valnet believes that microorganisms show no resistance (have no immunity) to essential oils. This may not be altogether true, but certainly whatever immunity they may have is minimal. Essential oils reliably inhibit microorganisms, destroying them either outright or eventually as the inhibition is prolonged. Essential oil results are achieved without the toxicity associated with chemicals and antibiotics, without contributing to tolerance or adaptation of the microbe, and without promoting secondary infections as happens with antibiotics.

The superiority of essential oils is also demonstrated by their versatility, both in application and in their simultaneous, multilevel effects, their safety, and their innate homeostatic intelligence. By direct and indirect contact, essential oils have two modes of action: while inhibiting the microbe, improving the terrain, and sparing supporting beneficial microorganisms, essential oils enhance natural immunity and increase the body's electromagnetic field. By contrast, antibiotics offer only one direct-contact mode of action, in the process of which they typically create harmful side-effects: damage to the terrain, destruction of innocent beneficial bacteria and flora along with the offending microbe, suppression of the body's own natural immunological response, and reduction of its surrounding electromagnetic field.

Essential oils also possess antiviral properties—another advantage they have over antibiotics, which have no effect on viruses. More insidious than bacteria, viruses actually invade and commandeer our own body cells and are therefore more difficult to combat. The antiviral effects of certain essential oils, such as tea tree, garlic, clove, geranium, cinnamon, thyme, black pepper, lavender, and eucalyptus, long observed experientially, have quickly gained experimental verification as well. Scientific tests show lavender and geranium to be particularly effective against herpes virus types. Russian scientific studies have shown the *in vitro* effectiveness of three more types of eucalyptus (*E. viminalis, E. macarthuri,* and *E. dalrypleana*) against two strains of influenza virus. Meanwhile, in Switzerland, antiviral preparations have been developed featuring essential oils (e.g., black pepper) and isolated terpenes. Positive research reports on the antiviral effects of black pepper oil have also been forthcoming from Germany and China.

Essential oils (and their aromatic hydrosols) safely and successfully treat disease and infection by combating pathogenic microbes, restoring healthy terrain, and stimulating body immunity. The parasiticidal effects of essential oils upon worms, lice, mites, crabs, and one-cell organisms are also well-documented. Too, they stimulate antitoxin action against not only insect bites and stings but also chemical poisons, such as drugs and alcohol. Essential oils are autoimmune stimulants and regulators that enhance *phagocytosis,* "eating by a cell"—the process by which various kinds of body cells ingest, and thereby destroy or deactivate, foreign particles such as bacteria or pollutants.

The marvelously complex immunological system of the human body releases a host of defenders that perform a multitude of protective defense manuevers. The phagocytic index includes several types of white blood cells (leukocytes) known by different names (neutrophils, T-cells, etc.) as well as microphages, macrophages, reticuloendothelial cells, lymphocytes, and other cells found plentifully in the liver, spleen, and lymph. Then there are the autoimmune antibodies: smart protein molecules synthesized by the body to cope specifically with virtually every conceivable potential antigen (foreign invader), including bacteria and viruses; fungi; pollen and dust allergens; insect venom; drugs and synthetic chemicals; foods; and foreign tissue from organ transplants, blood transfusions, and injections. These antibodies are a primary defense against cancer and allergies, and they provide both temporary and permanent immunity, as in cases of mumps and measles.

A transcending aspect of the body's self-defense involves electromagnetic energy and the otherwise metaphysical concept of *ether*, "life energy." Ether has been known by many names in different times and places, usually without specific attention given to its several grades: prana and kundalini (Hindu), chi (China), tumo (Tibet), bioplasma (USSR), vital fluid (medieval alchemy), quintessence or mumia (Paracelsus), eloptic energy (Galen Hieronymous), animal magnetism (Anton Mesmer), odic light force (Baron von Reichenbach), vital force (Dr. Samuel Hahnemann), orgone energy (Wilhelm Reich), biocosmic energy, X-force, mitogenic rays, psychotronic energy, and so on. Ether is visible as the aura—the etheric, electromagnetic force field shown by Kirlian photography—that surrounds and interpenetrates the dense, physical body, vitalizing, innervating, energizing, shielding, and protecting it. This "etheric double," so called because it is contoured to the more material physical form, is the intermediary link between the astral and physical bodies. Sustained malefic disturbances in this etheric sheath, caused by physical, atmospheric, environmental, physiological, or psychological means, can lead to ill-health and disease. Beneficial influences engender and foster glowing physical and psychological health.

Essential oils lend themselves to the promotion of the etheric or vital body and thus to psycho-physiological health, particularly by topical application or by inhalation and consequent olfactory nerve transmission. Healing touch—i.e., massage—directly magnifies the aura, even more so when performed with essential oils. The electromagnetic activity of essential oils can be demonstrated by the "Kirlian effect" shown by Kirlian photography. Plants capture the photo-electromagnetic energy of the sun— the single most powerful source of etheric energy in our planetary system, and the sole giver of life and master healer—converting, by their cellular and enzymatic action, the sun's life energy into biochemical energy, and actually condensing "soulful essence" from a spiritual force. The essential oil harbors this biochemical energy and essence.

Etheric or life energy is conducted throughout every cell, tissue, and organ of the physical body by blood circulation and transmitted along nerve pathways, especially the central nervous system. The etheric and astral bodies have centers or "organs" (chakras) that correspond to the ductless or endocrine glands, from which such energy is organized and emanates. Near the thymus gland, the master gland of the immune system, is one such chakra location establishing a link between physical and supraphysical functioning bodies. The etheric, hence metaphysical, effects of essential oils have spiritual implications, which is why aromatics has been vital to religious, liturgical, and meditative rituals and services.

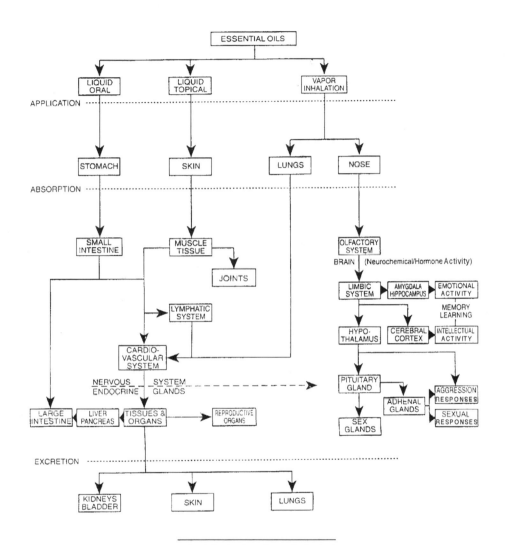

*Physiological and Psychological
Pathways for Essential Oils*

# 3

# Smell and the Psychology of Scent

## THE EVOLUTIONARY ROLE OF OLFACTION

One of the oldest, most primitive senses we possess, smell is presumably patterned after the kind of rudimentary chemical communication and discriminative skills first developed and exhibited by simpler, fundamental, single-cell life forms. Smell remained until very recently the most mysterious of senses, perhaps because in man's sensory development and perception, smell no longer plays the vital role it once did—and still does in other animals—having been lately superseded (in evolutionary terms) by the more advanced senses of hearing and sight. Our sense of smell is less prominent principally because our vertical spine provides the ability to stand erect and maintain an upright posture, from which we are more able to see and hear beyond the sensory range of smell. Yet, evaluated on its own merits, smell is as relevant and significant to the complete human experience as it has ever been.

The sense of smell is considerably less conspicuous than the physical organ with which it is identified—the nose. Yet, even for the nose itself, smell is a secondary, ancillary function, the primary function of the nose being to simultaneously channel, heat, and filter air and thereby provide life-giving oxygen to the lungs. The nose does this by its baffled structure, well supplied with nasal hairs and mucous membranes (epithelium). Although there are some 5 to 10 million scent-detecting olfactory cells positioned in the olfactory epithelium atop the nasal cavity within the nose, these cells are but a small contingent of the entire nasal mucous membrane, which is mostly non-olfactory, respiratory epithelium. (Nasal mucus provides a line of defense against invading bacteria, which are subjected to counteracting chemicals found in the mucus.) To further place this in relative perspective, one need only compare human olfactory cells with those of other animals for whom smell is an essential, indeed preeminent, sense. The rabbit has an estimated 100 million olfactory cells with a ready and constant turnover of new neuron cells emerging from basal cells within a few days. In humans and in other animals, scent detector cells have an extraordinary ability to replenish themselves, presumably in response to environmental exposure; i.e., damage or exhaustion. Indeed, the neurons in the human olfactory epithelium (mucous membrane) are the only neurons of the brain known to be capable of regeneration by basal cells. The regeneration rate says something about the relative importance of smell to each animal. Every 30 to 40 days completely new neurons appear in the human nose, a rate of replacement far too slow for the rabbit, whose very survival, unlike that of a human being, depends upon smell.

The dachshund has some 125 million olfactory cells and the sheepdog nearly twice that number, but since the receptive power and capacity of these cells increases exponentially, 220 million olfactory cells give the sheepdog a sense of smell approximately a million times more acute than that of a human. The bloodhound's sense of smell is 3 million times more sensitive or acute than is man's. Consequently, a smart tracking hound with a sharp nose can follow a scent trail several days old or even older, depending upon the quarry and environmental conditions. In *The Lives of a Cell*, author Lewis Thomas, one of America's most talented and distinguished physicians and medical researchers, presents twenty-nine essays of remarkable observations, some of which further illustrate the power and importance of smell in nature. He notes that ants can distinguish between themselves and other ants, leaving trails that can be followed by their own colony but not by other ants. Certain predator ants have, however, adaptively modified this ability to sense the trails of the other species that the predators routinely enslave. After tracking the unsuspecting victims to their nest, the invading predator ants then discharge odorants that panic and confuse their victims, whose capture soon follows. Although decidedly inferior to that of other animals (except perhaps other primates and most birds, which also have a relatively poor sense of smell), man's sense of smell is yet surprisingly strong, being able to detect hundreds—potentially thousands—of odors in very tiny amounts—e.g., a single molecule of bell pepper in a trillion molecules of air. The average person can smell a few sulfurous molecules of butyl mercaptan, and most people can detect minute amounts of musk. The musky odor of steroids is highly detectable, especially by women. Exaltolide is one synthetic steroid acutely perceptible to women but rarely to men. Probably owing to their excretion of formic acid, we can easily smell ants; thus *pismire* is a descriptive synonym for ant.

The millions of human olfactory cells are sensitive to some 10,000 different chemicals, by which a trained human nose can readily learn to distinguish several hundred odors. The ability of modern perfumery's professional "noses," who select from thousands of fragrance ingredients, is an example. Recently, the Los Angeles Department of Water and Power began utilizing a six-member team of "water sniffers" to improve the quality of city tap water. "The team has validated the scientific industry's claim that, in some cases, the human sense of smell is much more sensitive than any piece of equipment," reports Bruce Keubler, the department's director of water quality. Specially trained at UCLA to detect the kinds of odors and tastes that signal incipient water contamination by various chemicals, wastes, and dead or living organisms, the team serves "like an early warning system," according to Keubler. Actually, olfactory cell training (as occurs with tracking dogs) is common in nature. Repeated exposure to tiny doses of the same odorant prompts greater smell acuity, suggesting that smell receptors may be added to or by the existing cells, or that new cells with that particular receptor emerge during the training process. Olfactory training is part of the rehabilitory process for people suffering from anosmia—an inability to smell. In his book, Dr. Thomas reports that minnows, which recognize members of their own species by smell, have been taught to recognize phenol and to distinguish it from *p*-chlorophenol, in minute concentrations of five parts per billion. Eels have been likewise trained to smell just a few molecules of phenylethyl alcohol. By nature, eels, like salmon, somehow remember the odor of the waters in which they were hatched thereby later enabling them to return for spawning. Attached electrodes in the olfactory bulbs of salmon will fire when the olfactory epithelium is exposed to the salmon's original spawning water, whereas water from other sources elicits no response.

## The Olfactory System and Odor Perception

The human nose actually contains multiple independent systems or structures that in particular ways are chemically responsive to odor molecules (odorants). Two of these, the *terminal nerve* and the *septal nerve*, are least important. Although little is actually known of their structure and function, their potential response to odorants is uncertain if not doubtful. A third, the *trigeminal nerve*, responds to odorants by its common chemical sense—a generic, fundamental response to bases, acids, and other compounds—from nerve-ending branches that extend into the nose. Also known as the fifth or trifacial nerve, it is the largest cranial nerve and functions dually as the chief sensory nerve of the head and face and as the motor nerve for the muscles of mastication. Branches of the trigeminal nerve extending into the mouth and eyes provide, respectively, some taste sensitivity and response to airborne irritants. It too is of far less importance than the main olfactory system, but the trigeminal nerve does retain its fundamental odor response even after smell loss caused by damage to the primary olfactory system, thus providing a kind of electrochemical response that, while not really smell, is otherwise valuable in differentiating sensory impulses.

## Anatomy and Physiology of the Primary Olfactory System

As mentioned, besides the respiratory epithelium, the nose contains the *olfactory epithelium*, an area of special mucous membrane located at the roof of the inner nasal cavity. *Olfactory nerves*, neurons connected to the olfactory bulb located above the epithelium, protrude into the epithelium and project clusters of *olfactory cilia*—microscopic "hair" endings at the tip of each tiny nerve, designed to meet incoming odorants. (We are reminded that the human olfactory system has an estimated 10 million neurons, with at least 20 million cilia clusters or hair endings, surrounded by supporting cells.) Odorants entering the nose penetrate and dissolve into the mucus, where they encounter the cilia-tipped olfactory neurons located in the epithelium. The neurons respond to the submicroscopic particles of the odorant, triggering electrical nerve transmissions to the olfactory bulb. The nerve signal entering the bulb then travels along the olfactory tract into the brain.

Despite currently rapid progress in olfactory research, it remains unknown exactly how olfactory cells are fired by an odorant or how an odorant molecule impressed upon the olfactory epithelium is recognized and transduced (translated) into a nerve impulse. Odor molecules are chemically quite small. It seems that molecular geometry (i.e., size and especially shape or configuration) lends each odorant its own fragrance, uniquely determined by its geometric conformation of atoms and their bond angles. It may be that *osmic frequencies* —the special vibrations of atoms or atom groups within the odorant molecule (or the entire odorant molecule's own vibrational "song")—are another component of olfactory response if not the actual source of odor. Osmic frequencies may help explain the phenomena of subliminal smell or the subtle etheric and psychological responses to scents.

The most accepted hypothesis is that olfactory neurons contain on their cilia specific receptors for various odorants. That is, specific receptors within each cell fitted to respond to specific odorant molecules—a kind of "shape-matching" similar to the way in which the body designs antibodies to match individual antigens. This may involve "primary odor" receptors within different olfactory cells, capable of interpreting combinations. So far, such receptors are unidentified, and, unlike primary colors or tastes, the primary odors are as yet unnamed, although proponents of the shape-matching theory have suggested that seven classes of molecules produce seven basic odors: musky, flowery, pepperminty, etherlike, camphoraceous, pungent, and putrid. Based upon what we know, it is assumed that a given odorant stimulates a subset of primary receptors, causing a specific neural firing pattern that registers within the olfactory bulb and allows identification of the detected odorant. The specificity of odorant to receptor shape-matching is illustrated by lab experiments with carvone, a ketone constituent of essential oils that has two identical but mirror-image (stereoisomer) forms: *d*-carvone and *l*-carvone. The first smells of caraway; the second, of spearmint. Neural processing is able to distinguish the two, as demonstrated by those people who are particularly anosmic ("smell-blind") to one carvone scent but not to the other. Each carvone, therefore, matches and activates a different receptor.

## The "Dominose Effect"

If there is a physical key to the mystery of olfaction it may be found among proteins or enzymes that are instrumental to the molecular biology or biochemistry of olfaction. In recent years several proteins have been discovered in the olfactory cilia wherein specific receptors react to specific odorants. In 1990, scientists at Johns Hopkins University in Baltimore announced the discovery of yet another link in the biochemical chain reaction that occurs in the olfaction process: a chemical enzyme involved in amplifying the information presented by an odorant. The research is described by biologist Dr. Randall Reed in the then-current issue of *Science* journal. Evidently, protein enzymes are key participants in the olfactory system's signaling relay scheme. Starting from the probable assumption that the way olfaction sensory cells discriminate among odors is determined by molecules upon their surface, whereby certain molecules react with certain chemicals, here is how the "dominose effect" involving the newly identified proteins and enzyme is thought to happen:

1. Entering the system, one of the 10,000 chemical compounds (odorants) detectable by human smell finds its corresponding receptor molecule, and the odorant is bound to that specific receptor by what scientists now call odorant-binding protein (OBP). Concentrated in the Steno's gland located in the lateral wall of the nasal cavity, OBP is released into nasal mucus via the gland's duct extending toward the tip of the nose and is thereby distributed throughout the rest of the nose, where it can more readily engage inhaled odorants, binding and transporting them within the mucus.

2. After binding contact with the odorant, the receptor activates another kind of protein that sequentially activates the enzyme, amplifying the signal received. The sensory cell reacts to the surface encounter with the odorant by releasing thousands of molecules of the newly identified enzyme.

3. These enzyme molecules in turn activate chemical nerve "messengers" that cause the neurons attached to the sensory cells to transmit signals to the brain via the olfactory bulb and tract.

4. The brain interprets the nerve transmission signals originating from the specific sensory cell as evidence that a particular odorant has been encountered.

This seemingly detailed account is necessarily a simplified, abbreviated version of the more involved biochemical process that actually occurs. Complex odors may, of course, activate various sensory cells, sending the brain numerous signals in combination, which it must process and identify. Dr. Reed confidently claims that all but one of the biochemicals in the olfaction process have now been ascertained, that one being the all-important receptor molecule that presumably first encounters the odor molecule on the surface of the olfaction sensory cell. Since the nose is sensitive to thousands of different chemicals, it is expected that a matching number of different biochemical receptor molecules must also exist, but Dr. Reed expects that their differences will be very slight and optimistically predicts that after the first of them are discovered, the rest will be quickly found. Still, conclusive explanations for olfaction remain scarce, while new discoveries also raise questions requiring more complex and elusive answers.

## Pheromones—the Hidden Persuaders

How it is that a bloodhound can track a shoe-clad man across open ground, even when the scent trail is days old and cluttered with other conflicting scents, illustrates the power of something else as remarkable as the dog's olfactory gifts: pheromones. The word *pheromone* derived from the Greek *pherein*, "to carry," and *hormon*, "to excite," aptly describes biochemical molecules that do indeed "carry excitement." By spraying and rubbing, animals either secrete or excrete pheromones to transmit a myriad of powerful signals that define status, rank, and sexual and social identification, and that mark territorial boundaries and trails. Because they affect sexual, aggressive, and other physical behaviors, pheromones can be used to confuse, revulse, or frighten enemies as well as to attract and beguile new or familiar friends. Natural human odor once served similar purposes and still does to some extent by the pheromones excreted in our sweat. Mammals, including humans and other primates, release pheromones from specialized apocrine glands. These olfactory signals communicate information about our physical health, sexual status, and emotional changes. Pheromones secreted by the apocrine glands of human feet can linger for as long as two weeks. Every barefoot step, leaving as little as four-billionths of a gram of odoriferous sweat substance, appears like a road map to a bloodhound; indeed, that minute amount is enough to penetrate shoes and be detectable by a good tracking hound.

At the Monell Chemical Senses Center in Philadelphia, the research laboratory where the aforementioned carvone experiment was conducted, Dr. George Preti has discovered the molecular ingredient that gives axillary (underarm) perspiration its characteristic odor. Bound to a peptide, the molecule is released by the sweat glands. Initially too large to be nasally detected, the water-soluble molecule must first be split from the peptide by skin bacteria to become smell detectable. It may or may not be a pheromonal molecule. The continuing analysis of pheromones in other primates began decades ago. In 1971, it was reported that male-attractant, short-chain aliphatic compounds (acids) appear in the vaginal secretions of female monkeys responding to estradiol. Whether these and other suspected pheromones have socio-sexual behavioral significance among primates, whose sense of smell is not acute, is still under investigation.

## Human Pheromones and the Vomeronasal Organ

There are numerous reasons to infer the active presence of human pheromones. First, we know that prehistoric man and more recent primitive peoples have relied heavily on their sense of smell for survival. The human anatomical evidence—apocrine glands, specifically located hair patches and moisture areas, and skin folds designed for controlled bacterial growth and activity—also suggests the existence of pheromones. But perhaps the most convincing anatomical evidence is a recently rediscovered vomeronasal organ in humans.

The *vomeronasal organ* (VNO), a separate sensory nasal structure distinct from the primary olfactory system, is located low in the nose of animals that have it. In most terrestrial vertebrates it responds to pheromones. Activated when the mouth opens, it detects large, nonvolatile molecules (such as pheromones) that are less capable or incapable of airborne travel or of interaction with the olfactory epithelium. Thought to be vestigial in humans, this organ is how animals detect sexually intimate pheromonal messages. Knowing that nature retains nothing that is useless, we must deduce that the vomeronasal organ located in the tip of the human nose operates in a similar way. Indeed, recent research at the universities of

Colorado and Utah shows that at least 90 percent of human beings still possess the vomeronasal organ by which they respond biochemically and bioelectrically to the presence of chemical pheromones.

First described nearly 300 years ago by a Dutch military surgeon, the cone-shaped vomeronasal organ appears in each nostril as a tiny pit located at the bottom of the septal wall that divides the nose. Sometimes visible to the naked eye, each VNO pit may vary in size from nearly a tenth of an inch across to as small as a microscopic one-hundredth of an inch. Actually the organ's opening, the pit leads into a tenths of an inch long duct lined with unusual neuron receptor cells. These cells somehow communicate sensory information to the hypothalamus and limbic system structures of the brain, probably via the many connecting neurons surrounding the vomeronasal organ.

Most known pheromones are simple molecules, active in extremely low concentrations. Eight or ten carbon atoms in a chain are enough to chemically transmit precise and compelling behavioral instructions. They are classified into two general categories: *signaling pheromones*, which incite ready and immediate behavioral responses from the recipient, and *primer pheromones*, which trigger complex physiological activity such as glandular hormonal activity. Signaling pheromones of animals are highly involved in sexual reproduction encounters. Primer pheromones regulate puberty and ovulation, among other events. Ovulation or the onset of female puberty in animals can either be accelerated by exposure to male pheromones or delayed by the pheromonal presence of other females. Inversely, the sexual maturation rate or onset of puberty for male animals can be accelerated by female pheromonal stimuli or delayed by the presence of male stimuli. Lacking male stimuli, the estrus (female sexual) cycle is suppressed and often synchronized among female animals living as a group. The same behavior is exhibited by humans. Women synchronize their menstrual periods when they live among other women. For example, the observed synchronization of menstrual periods in all-girls dormitories is caused by pheromonal exchange (trading or pooling) of instructional information transmitted in human sweat, particularly axillary (armpit) secretions, signaling synchronous menstruation.

In humans, male pheromonal odors also influence the female menstrual cycle. Menstrual regularity is promoted by male companionship, and female puberty is accelerated when women live near men. Perhaps in keeping with the greater acidity of male perspiration, male pheromones are more musky than are female pheromones. When exposed to musk, women ovulate more readily and show more sexual arousal. A woman's sense of smell significantly heightens during ovulation, usually peaking at midcycle. (Heightened smell apparently correlates to elevated estrogen levels.) With perfume ingredients, especially those like civet or musk, perfumers seek to mimic sexually charged pheromones, especially the musk-like human odors particularly strong in men. For example, sandalwood's scent appeal may be due to its chemical similarity to androsterol, a male pheromone. Secreted in the saliva of male boars, the sex pheromones androstenone and androstenol have a powerfully compelling mating affect upon sows. Both pheromones are also secreted by human apocrine glands located in the genital and axillary areas. A fairly ubiquitous molecule, androstenone can be found in human saliva as well as in underarm sweat; it also appears in pork products and some vegetables. Yet, an estimated 40 to 50 percent of the United States population is "smell-blind" to it.

Owing to a variety of mediating and mitigating physiological, psychological, and social factors, the effects of pheromones on human behavior are somewhat less compelling and dramatic than they are upon animal behavior. But subtle and subliminal olfactory responses to pheromones and other biochemical odorants nonetheless alter human behavior and, to some extent, human judgement by affecting us emotionally and physiologically—which is to also say instinctively. These effects are of great interest not only to the flavor and fragrance industries but also to others who seek new means and opportunities to modify personal and social human behavior.

## Olfaction and Immunology

Experiments at Monell Chemical Senses Center, revealing how a rodent's odor is linked to its immunology, demonstrate the physical law of opposites attracting. Like other animals, a rat seeks a mate with a different immunological type, indeed the most different, presumably for creating a wider range of immunology for the species' survival. The rat identifies the different immunotype mate by smell. We already know that olfactory communication is crucial to symbiotic relationships between different species; e.g., the crab and sea anemone, the anemone and damsel fish. Symbiosis—the mutually dependent, beneficial partnership between two organisms—predates and anticipates more complex immunological sensing as a survival technique. When watching the rodent search for a mate, we are observing the convergence and interrelationship of olfaction and immunology, both involving biochemistry. It may be that immunological responses, such as the development of antibodies, evolved with or from symbiotic sensing featuring smell. Symbiotic sensing follows the dichotomous principle of attraction/repulsion, using odors and olfaction to attract symbionts and to repel predatory parasites and adversaries. As in symbiosis, smell and immunology are linked, correlative mechanisms in the differentiation or discrimination of self from nonself. Half the genes that develop the immune system of a child come from the father, half from the mother. During embryonic and postnatal development, the child learns its first biological lesson in self-tolerance by making the immunological adjustment between the two halves.

There is a large, as yet undetermined number of olfactory receptor genes. Likewise, one's personal odor is genetically programmed. Despite racial or ethnic grouping, which impart common odor and olfaction traits to the individual, personal body odor is as unique as fingerprints. Even identical twins, presumably having the same genetic makeup, can be distinguished by body odor, owing to each's body chemistry, bacterial synthesis of fatty acids, diet, and other personal habits. Your individual odor may vary according to changing psycho-physiological states, but it remains nonetheless your own.

Nobel Prize-winning immunologist Niels K. Jerne interprets the human search for a mate as essentially a search for immune system compatibility, more specifically for someone of the opposite sex with a compatible (suitable, not necessarily similar) human leukocyte antigen system (HLA). Not only does sexual odor-olfactory communication occur among humans, clinical observations indicate that couples who are odor-incompatible have unsuccessful relationships. The necessary olfactory and immunological adjustments between prospective mates are fundamental, not cosmetic. During sexual intimacy thousands, if not millions, of cellular substances—skin and hair material, saliva, sweat, sexual fluids, and germs—are exchanged. This is a major immunological challenge to both persons' systems. By touching, and especially by kissing, we intimately and immediately exchange not only pheromonal messages via the vomeronasal organ but also bacteria and cellular information testing our immunological compatibility. Artificially scented modern man believes he has buried his natural, genetically designed odor along with his primitive past. Modern woman, especially, uses more kinds of acquired fragrances, perfumes, and deodorants to establish individual and social identity and status, to allure males by increasing her range of attractiveness through volatile airborne scents. Today's sophisticated scents do indeed appeal to and stimulate elaborate emotions rather than primal urges and basic instinct, and for that purpose manufactured, acquired scents are more effective than our more primitively direct natural odor. But ultimately and intimately, pheromones and other odoriferous bodily secretions are the scents that matter in subliminal olfactory and immunological compatibility, and which no acquired scent can substitute for or permanently disguise.

# OSMOLOGY—THE STUDY OF SMELL

Osmics, the science of odors, and osmology (Greek: *osme*, "smell") contribute, among other things, valuable observations and useful terminology to the understanding of smell and taste. The following is a short glossary of basic terms used to classify and describe various smell and taste conditions:

> *Anosmia*—lack of or inability to smell
> *Cacosmia*—foul smell
> *Dysosmia*—dysfunctional distorted smell
> *Hyperosmia*—increased ability to smell
> *Hyposmia*—reduced ability to smell
> *Osmatic*—acute sense of smell
> *Osmesis*—smelling
> *Osphresis*—sense of smell
> *Parosmia*—distorted smell of imaginary odors
> *Ageusia*—loss of taste
> *Dysgeusia*—abnormal taste
> *Gustation*—sense of taste
> *Hypogeusia*—reduced taste

There are numerous causes of what can be permanent or temporary abnormalities within these categories, particularly anosmia (loss of smell). Sinusitis, allergies, nasal polyps, tissue damage, and head trauma (injuries) are the most common. Also, surgical or toxic side-effects or exposure to drugs or medical therapies, nerve or endocrine disorders, and nutritional deficiencies, such as a lack of vitamin A or of the mineral element zinc and concurrent zinc-copper imbalance.

Anosmia, the loss of smell (also called *osnomia*), is not merely an aesthetic diminishment of life's pleasures afforded through taste and aroma, it is potentially hazardous as well. For example, the sensory detection of danger signals (fire smoke, gas leak fumes, bad food or water) is also reduced or lost. According to E. Douek, writing in *Perfumery: The Psychology and Biology of Fragrance*, anosmia is always associated with psychological depression paralleling the dullness of taste and smell. Although depression among the elderly may arise from many other concurrent social and psychological causes, the aged suffer most from anosmia as the sense of smell declines, like the other senses, with advancing years. (Our power of smell apparently peaks between the ages of twenty and forty.) Yet, research indicates that the osnomia of the elderly selectively occurs first with bad odors, whereas sensitivity to pleasant odors remains relatively normal even into the more advanced age of eighty or ninety years. Discounting any of the known or detectable physiological causes, is anosmia in the otherwise healthy elderly person a normal, natural development? (The same might be asked about other sensory decline.) Is it the expected consequence of a lifetime of abuse and exposure, despite the remarkably unique regenerative powers of olfaction cells? Have those elderly people who are selectively osnomic developed antiodorants designed to block recognition of malodors or defend against them? Do other elderly osnomics develop antiodorants that eventually block scent perception altogether? Dr. Susan Schiffman, professor of medical psychology in the psychiatry department at Duke University, confirms the apparent atrophy and selectivity of smell in the aged, citing that the average smell sensory threshold of people in their 70s is about eight times higher than the threshold of people in their 20s and that there is clearly more adaptation to odors among the elderly. Yet, their reduction in olfactory perception varies widely for different odor stimuli.

There is a distinction between selective anosmia—smell blindness to some or many odorants—and total anosmia, the complete loss of smell. Besides that gradually occurring in the aged, much if not most permanent anosmia, whether selective or total, is probably genetic in origin, perhaps owing to the lack of some protein or enzyme such as those now being identified. This might, of course, be more obvious in congenital cases of total anosmia.

Dysosmia (smell distortion) more usually means unpleasant smell perception, cacosmia, or parosmia. Douek observes that parosmia reveals psychological behavior: shyness and timidity in those who believe the unpleasant odor originates from themselves, paranoia in those who believe the odor emanates from others. We know that paranoid schizophrenics characteristically have a distorted sense of smell (as well as of taste and other senses) while also exuding a peculiar, unfamiliar odor themselves. Both concurrent abnormalities, of smell and odor, arise from a biochemical disturbance or imbalance. (Specifically, the strange odor of schizophrenics has been attributed to the secretion of trans-3-methylhexanoic acid in their sweat.) Perhaps their smell distorts actual existing odors, or detects new, strange, and ordinarily undetectable odors, or detects imaginary, nonexistent odors—or all three. One wonders too whether their unusual smell distortion (or recognition?) occurs in the nose or in the brain.

Douek notes that such "parosmic paranoia" accompanies suspicion of others and may lead to conspiratorial or even retaliatory behavior. He cites French king Louis XI, a notorious tyrant, as one example of this parosmic paranoid behavior. Sigmund Freud was among the first to note the relationship of smell disturbances or repression to mental illness. He also inferred the connection between smell (the nose) and sexuality (the sexual organs). Freud was also among the first to correctly diagnose schizophrenia as a biochemical disease amenable to chemical cure. Today's osmology, through olfactory research, could hold promise for the diagnosis, relief, or cure of many psychological illnesses by the correction of smell abnormalities and the use of odors. Just as smell abnormality is linked to depression and to anxiety, impaired smell may precede or coincide with mental, cognitive decline. Potential diagnostic treatment could include not just classic psychological ills (e.g., schizophrenia or manic depression) but also neuropsychiatric problems, such as Alzheimer's disease, for which odors may stimulate recall, brain chemicals and their transmission, and neural pathways, increasing awareness and orientation. Psychological illness has been successfully treated for centuries with aromatic oils. On the other side of the olfactory equation, smell has been a naturopathic diagnostic tool dating back to the ancient Greeks and Egyptians and to kinds of Oriental medicine still practiced today, whereby smell is used to detect diseases—schizophrenia, diabetes, infection, nutritional imbalances or deficiencies—that are revealed by the odors of breath, body, urine, or feces.

## A Matter of Taste

A plainer example of dysosmia is a rare metabolic disorder known as fish-odor syndrome (trimethylaminuria) caused by the absence of enzyme $n$-oxidase. Lacking this enzyme, people suffering this disorder cannot convert trimethylamine from choline found in eggs, beans, liver, and other foods. Consequently, to these people such foods may taste like rotten fish and impart a fishy odor to their saliva, sweat, and urine. That fish-odor syndrome could as easily be termed "fish-taste syndrome"—a case of dysgeusia, or abnormal taste—points up the close interrelationship between separate physiological systems. Taste abnormalities share many of the same causes as smell disorders, such as injuries, diseased states, and nutritional or biochemical deficiencies.

We are told that 80 percent—some say 90 percent—of taste is actually smell. Owing to the close proximity and often shared activity of the two systems, we fail to distinguish between their functions, instead mentally blending the real distinctions between taste, smell, flavor, and aroma just as we do when we eat. The interaction between taste and smell commences with the link between aroma and appetite. Just as food aroma enhances appetite, hunger increases sensitivity to food aromas. Conversely, satiation (after eating) diminishes smell sensitivity. (Obesity reduces smell acuity owing to a chronic, static satiation response; the body is already overfed.) The selective activation of digestive enzymes is partly triggered by food odors, but taste has the leading role in digestive decisions and makes its own contribution to the personal health and safety of the organism.

Gustation, the sense of taste, has received far less attention from the scientific community than has olfaction. Other than the pain response of physical feeling (touch), taste is the only separate sensory system that is fully developed at birth. Like touch, taste is a fundamental survival apparatus—more so than smell. The development of smell, while important to the survival of the individual organism, is even more essential for the perpetual preservation of the species. Taste is strictly an individual preservation response mechanism. Like smell, taste operates, albeit in more primitive fashion, along the same dichotomous either/or principle of attraction/repulsion, which also governs the responses of physical feeling or touch to stimuli of pain and pleasure.

Taste has four qualities or criteria for discrimination—sweet, salty, sour, and bitter—strategically located, respectively, from the tip to the back of the tongue. Smell allows us to elaborate upon those four basic, simple responses to better enjoy the flavors and aromas of food and to make the complex choices and evaluations involved in the omnivorous diet of a complex organism. For simpler creatures on a virtually restricted, less varied monodiet, whether carnivorous or herbivorous, such choices and evaluations are less useful or critical. Immediately at birth, human babies like sweets and dislike bitter substances. This is an instinctive response based on attraction to substances that are safe and healthful (sweet) and repulsion of those that are harmful or even poisonous (bitter). In our own vernacular we reveal this elementary response when describing events, circumstances, or even people as bitter or sweet. Both smell and taste produce fundamental good/bad responses revealed in our language, for example, when we say that something or someone "stinks" (is bad). A sweet deal is good, as is the sweet smell of success. In *gustation* we see the root word *gust*, "to relish," from which derives *gusto*, which has the same meaning. *Disgust* means literally "to nauseate" and expresses feelings of strong aversion, loathing, or repugnance. Someone or something we find offensive, abhorrent, or worthy of our hatred is described as odious, meaning that we dislike the bad smell.

Smell, taste, and touch represent our gut reactions, but taste and touch are the foremost arbiters of what is in the physical organism's best survival interests. Although taste hasn't the regenerative powers of smell (taste buds on the tongue cannot replace themselves) the importance of taste is revealed by its resiliency: even when the several different nerves that supply or serve the throat, palate, and tongue are severed or anesthetized, taste cannot be denied.

## Motherhood and Infancy

Female olfaction fluctuates more dramatically with hormonal changes. While a woman's sense of smell perception heightens during ovulation, her smell is relatively dulled soon after conception and throughout the first trimester of pregnancy before once again becoming osmatic. This is an instinctive sequence mechanism. First, it restrains sexual intercourse, prevents ovulation, and ensures pregnancy or reproductive efforts once conception is accomplished, suspending the menses and preventing pheromonal interference with pregnancy. Later it heightens smell sensitivity for the protection

71

of the more developed fetus, whose demands increase after the earlier embryonic stage of pregnancy.

The smell distortions (dysosmia) of pregnant women are typically osmatic or hyperosmic. Many odors, even familiar or favorite scents, can become repellent or too strong. Unsurprisingly, an aversion to certain food odors and tastes often occurs simultaneously, commonly including fish, meat, tobacco, and coffee. Food aversion is a natural, primary child protection mechanism, as is sudden nausea or morning sickness. When they occur they are naturally necessary. Such aversions are most frequently temporary or persist until childbirth; some can be permanent if they are reinforced by emotional association.

Olfactory communication among humans has its origins in our past and present animal nature. Among animals, lasting bonds are immediately established between mother and offspring. Young animals and their mothers exchange odor signals that alternately stimulate and perpetuate maternal and nursing instincts and also enable them to identify and locate each other and the home site. As with other animals, there is a powerful olfactory bond between human mother and child, beginning in pregnancy. This bond is greatly strengthened by breast feeding and lasts well into childhood and beyond.

Virtually from birth, an infant can discriminate his own mother's odor from the odors of other mothers. This osmic identification is mutual. With her eyes closed, a mother can readily identify her own baby by smell. Likewise, there is a similar touch bond. In a study coauthored by members of Hebrew University and the Shaare Zedek Medical Center in Jerusalem, under tightly controlled experimental conditions, 70 percent of mothers tested could identify their own newborns by feeling the back of the infants' hands. (The research was reported in the January, 1992 journal issue of *Developmental Psychology* by coauthor Marsha Kaitz, psychology professor at the university.) Each participant's eyes and nose were covered by a heavy cotton scarf to block sight and smell, and only the right hand of each infant was exposed to the mothers' touch. Most participating mothers said they identified their own children by the texture and temperature of the infants' hands. Significantly, all the participating women had breastfed their babies, once again demonstrating the superior bonding effect of breast feeding and breast milk itself. A sweet, perfectly formulated infant food, breast milk has more than just the known nutritional advantages over bottled milk formulas.

Among its other benefits, breast feeding promotes superior immunology, oral and sensory development, and the psychological health of the child.

## Family, Friends, Foreigners

Infants have other very definite olfactory preferences, dispelling the long-held misconception that smell preferences are entirely learned, acquired by cultural or social mimicry and training. Predictably, their preferences are highest for familiar odors, beginning with those of their mothers. Humans can distinguish the odor differences between and among themselves, i.e., their family, friends, and strangers. Preferences for perfumes, fragrances, food aromas, and other natural or environmental odors reflect real differences of odor perception and odor transmission between ethnic and racial groups. While the odor of each individual is unique, there is a significant commonality of odor and odor perception within these groups, owing to genetically determined olfactory anatomy, such as olfaction receptors, and skin types (and consequently bacteria synthesis and biochemistry). Humans can smell and be smelled by other members of their genetic group. The subconsciously identifiable odor of a human ethnic or racial group transmits that group's immunologic and genetic information, fostering group identity and maximizing preservation. Cultural, social, and environmental factors will reinforce or mitigate that information to some small degree.

On April 8, 1991, in her "Response of the scientific community to olfactory power and potential" to Summit 2000: Preparing For The First Global Civilization, Dr. Susan Schiffman of Duke University reported that improved communication and reduced personal, physical distance between people of different nationalities results from their mutual familiarity with each's culturally produced odors. She produced her conclusions by experimentally exposing a group of people from multinational and multiracial backgrounds to clothing, fragrances, foods, candles, and incense gathered from different countries and displayed on a center table for smell examination. Actually, the procedure is not unlike the kind of international trade and market activity already occurring in the world. Although there are other plausible explanations for the group's behavior, Dr. Schiffman suggests that deliberate exposure to multicultural odors (genetic or otherwise) will promote toleration of cultural diversity and world peace, and that society should begin exposing youngsters to foreign cultural odors to increase their acceptance of others whose scent differs from their own. Some people regard

Dr. Schiffman's proposal as progressive, altruistic, and even visionary. Some people see in it another social engineering threat designed to undermine natural family bonds and cultural ties and to erase national identities—a One World Osphresis for a New World Odor. Others dismiss the notion of teaching the world to smell in perfect harmony as simplistic utopianism, noting that such efforts are better conducted by God, nature, and spontaneous social evolution. Similarly concerned viewpoints emerge in discussion and debate over subliminal "environmental fragrancing" and other scientific objectives involving olfaction, which will be explored in a later chapter. Above all, by reviewing and examining the ideas, opinions, and experiments of researchers like Dr. Schiffman, we learn the seriousness of the scientific community's interest in olfaction and how that interest is at variance with aromatherapy.

# OLFACTION AND THE BRAIN

The path of an odorant leads into the nose, into the primary and ancillary olfactory systems, and so directly into the brain. Indeed, the olfactory nerves extend directly into the brain—or you might say that the brain extends outward into the nose. The olfactory neurons meet cells in the olfactory bulb that help chemically convert the odorant signal, sending their relay output of the signal directly to the limbic system, in far less time than we have taken to explain the process. Smell is the only sense that has this direct access and route to the brain; taste, touch, sight, and hearing arrive at the limbic system through indirect pathways.

## The Limbic System

Also known as the "old brain" because of its more primitive function and earlier evolutionary development, the limbic system was originally called the *rhinencephalon*, the "smell brain." In the late nineteenth century it was renamed *le grand lobe limbique* by the French anatomist Broca, who observed that despite having an especially pronounced, well-developed limbic system, the dolphin has surprisingly little olfactory sense; hence the name's connotation of a suspended or limited function. Broca later identified the two coils of tissue (convolutions) included in the limbic system that are more specifically well developed in osmatic animals, such as the dog and fox.

Described by G. O. Watts in *Dynamic Neuroscience: Its Application to Brain Disorders*, the limbic system is a complex ring of brain structures and interconnected pathways arranged into fifty-three regions and thirty-five associated tracts. The limbic system and hippocampus together form a central switchboard to coordinate all sensory input (sights, sounds, smells) into a whole. The limbic system tends to evaluate sensory stimuli, especially those received by smell, taste, and touch, according to the dichotomous principle of attraction/repulsion (acceptance or rejection), which prevails on the emotional level of being (like vs. dislike) and on the physical level, where it is similarly interpreted as a basic choice between pleasure or pain, safety or danger, pursuit or avoidance. In the human limbic system (and the hypothalamus, to which it is closely related) we observe the intersection of emotional feelings and desires with physical needs and instincts. Together the limbic system and hypothalamus initiate and govern primitive and emotional drives—sex, thirst, hunger, etc.—evoking visceral and behavioral mechanisms and such "gut feeling" responses as rage, fear, sorrow, revulsion, physical affection, and sexual attraction. The pheromonal-sexual-olfactory connection takes place in the limbic-hypothalamic region of the brain. We can now see how and why smell relates to emotion: smell directly accesses the limbic system and hypothalamus, wherein instincts and biological emotions lie and the neurochemical/hormonal regulation of the body is controlled, and also accesses other parts of the brain, all involving memory, attention, and psychosomatic integration.

There is a parallel connection between olfaction and brain development. An undeveloped nasal bone is a signature of mental retardation. Each year in the United States, some 3,000 unfortunate babies are born anencephalic—that is, with a rare and deadly congenital defect that begets hopeless creatures kept alive, for a time, artificially. Missing most, if not all, of the brain cerebrum and cortex, the cerebellum, and the skin and bone covering, a baby with anencephaly is born without a brain. It is also born without a nose. Perhaps now we can better comprehend why the ancient art of physiognomy, which interprets the qualities of the mind through facial features, contours, and expressions, has long extolled the merits of the classic Roman nose (firm, straight, and strongly bridged) while also noting the meaningful diversity in nose shapes and sizes and reciprocal brain development among human beings.

Homolateral (same-side) brain-olfaction development is noticeable from the embryonic stage; the improper development of one brain hemisphere, left or right, will correspond to underdevelopment of the nasal cavity on the same side. The correlation between smell, nasal development, and human intelligence is well established and is displayed by the link between smell disorders and learning disabilities or mental illness. Moreover, just as prolonged or permanent sensory deprivation will lead to depression and atrophy of the other sensory organs and corresponding areas of the brain, smell deprivation—total anosmia—or the total reduction of odorous air will eventually contribute to brain degeneration from enervation and a lack of blood circulation.

## The Cerebrum

The surface of the human cerebrum, the large brain mass called the *cerebral cortex*, is a 2-millimeter-thick, densely packed, and highly interconnected mass of neuron cell bodies and dendrites. Although the cerebrum and cortex actually contain both gray and white matter, their predominantly gray color is attributable to that of the unsheathed neuron tissue; hence "gray matter" has become synonymous with intelligence. Other than the porpoise, no other organism has a cerebral cortex as large, as abundant with intricate convolutions (tissue coils, folds, and fissures), and as highly developed as man's. By all connotations, the cerebral cortex of the cerebrum is the highest part of the brain, directing voluntary motor functions and movements from head to toe and out to the extremities, and the sensory functions and movements of sight and hearing as well as speech. The cerebrum and cerebral cortex are organizationally divided into hemispheres. The left and right hemispheres are connected by the *corpus callosum*, a large nerve bundle or bridge (commissure) that allows the two hemispheres to communicate.

## The Brain Hemispheres

As recently as the nineteenth century, before commissurotomy, the surgical division of the hemispheres, was first performed in the late 1940s, it was thought that splitting the hemispheres would create two separate personalities. But other than preventing severe epileptic seizures from spreading from one side to the other (a benefit to some epileptics), commissurotomy otherwise prevented the hemispheres from communicating and transferring information.

76

Lately many fanciful and exaggerated claims have been made about "creative differences," even a "conceptual antagonism," that supposedly exists between the hemispheres. Although the hemispheres are of similar shape and appearance, it is true that they are not identical. Indeed, they are quite unalike in several important ways. But except by radical surgery, a real division does not exist. The right and left hemispheres are well integrated and are made highly cooperative by the corpus callosum, across which, as well as across other commissures or structures elsewhere in the brain, there is much "cross-talk." Regrettably, recent scientific efforts to distinguish the relative functions and distinctive attributes of the hemispheres have been tainted by competitive social ideas, trendy pop psychology, and romantic New Age notions that glorify the right brain while belittling the left brain almost as if each were a separate personality. By those popular portrayals, the left brain is boring, dull, pedestrian, rigidly restricted, and predictable. Conversely, we are told, the right brain is the deep, yet soaring fountain of intuitive creativity, wisdom, and enlightenment, which would (if not shackled by the fearfully inhibited, jealously oppressive left brain) transform each of us into a happily inspired and expressive genius—all of which is wonderfully absurd nonsense. The right brain is neither intuitive nor particularly creative, although it is aesthetically imaginative. Imagination and emotional feeling frequently masquerade as intuition, and the right brain is emotional. It is also irrational: the right brain cannot think. Language, culture, reading, writing, speech, and most physical skills—those things that distinguish human consciousness—reside almost exclusively in the left hemisphere. "The right side is a very stupid hemisphere," says Michael Gazzaniga, director of the Center for Neuroscience and professor of neurology and psychology at the University of California–Davis. "It's a very minor cognitive system. I don't even know [that] you could assign it an attitude. It might have some conditioned responses."

Whereas the left brain, the center of conscious cognition and rational thought, controls the expression of speech, the right brain is mute. When the hemispheres are surgically isolated, first by severing the corpus callosum nerve bridge, they function independently of one another. Alone, the irrational right hemisphere has little or no aptitude for verbal expression because it cannot perceive, obtain knowledge, or understand what is presented through the senses. A simplified, condensed account of a more complex lab experiment illustrates this fact.

When asked "What did you see?" after a projected picture of a spoon had been shown to her right brain (via her left field of vision), one commissurotomy patient replied, "Nothing." When shown a *Playboy* photo of a nude woman, the same patient giggled and blushed but still said she saw nothing. Asked why she was giggling, she could only reply, "Oh, doctor, you have some machine!" Later, when shown the same photo through her right visual field to her left brain, she immediately recognized why she had giggled and blushed. Previously, her right brain, responding emotionally, had registered her feelings, but the detached left brain's language center, where sensory input is identified, interpreted, and translated into words for speech, hadn't "seen" the *Playboy* photo.

Some 200 commissurotomy procedures have been performed since the 1960s, mostly to treat severe epilepsy. Most of the time, when both their eyes are open, the patients function normally. Sometimes, after brain surgery in which an entire hemisphere must be removed (e.g., to treat brain cancer) a human being will function surprisingly well because the remaining hemisphere compensates for the loss. It is possible that when necessary, the right hemisphere can assume some of the mental and physical skills of the left hemisphere. In one medical case, reported in 1966, a 47-year-old man's entire left hemisphere was surgically removed. Within a year after the operation, he had relearned how to eat, walk, manually help with the dishwashing, do simple arithmetic, and express himself verbally. It must be remembered that the left hemisphere is actually larger and heavier, is packed with more neurons, and shows more convolutions. The less complexly designed and developed right brain is not "neuron-rich" enough to manage the delicate, intricate functions of speech and hand movements; it has little capability for organized thought, analysis, reasoned speculation, or the other mental activities normally performed by the left brain.

## The Cerebrospinal or Central Nervous System (CNS)

The afferent and efferent nerves of the human body—respectively, all nerves carrying sensory impulses toward the CNS (brain and spine) and those nerves carrying impulses from the CNS to the muscles and glands—are cross-wired. The afferent and efferent nerves of the body's left side cross over to the right brain; the right side nerves cross over to the left brain. Of the two hemispheres, the left is nearly always dominant. And while one might expect that to be the situation for right-handed people, it is almost invariably true among left-handed people too, which may explain why there are so few of them. In fact, as few as 3 percent of people (an estimated 3 to 7 percent) are consistently left-handed, whereas nearly 70 percent are consistently right-handed. The rest perform different tasks with different hands; some perform the same tasks with either hand, but usually the right hand is more prominent. We are all ambidextrous to some extent, and "handedness" is not precisely defined. (There is "leggedness" also.) But, true ambidexterity—equal hand facility and ability in all things—is quite rare.

The nerves of the head go to both hemispheres of the cerebrum. That is why, for instance, stimulation of the auditory area in either hemisphere will create the sensation that sound is coming from both ears simultaneously. In many lower animals each eye is separately wired to only one hemisphere of the brain. In humans, the vision nerves are subdivided, as you can demonstrate for yourself in the following exercise:

Looking straight ahead with one eye closed, hold a pencil vertically in front of the open eye, dividing the field of vision into equal halves. Everything you see to the left of the pencil is received in the right hemisphere of the cerebral cortex; everything seen to the right of the pencil is received in the left hemisphere. Both eyes operate the same way. In short, the nerves for the left half of the vision field in both eyes are wired to the right hemisphere, and the nerves for the right half of the vision field in both eyes are wired to the left hemisphere. Thus, the field of vision of either eye or both eyes is equally and simultaneously represented to both sides of the brain— at least ideally. There is no sharp line of demarcation in each eye where the wiring abruptly begins and ends. Usually, the nerves "blend" in the middle of the eye, but one hemisphere may possibly receive a disproportionate share of reception from both eyes or even from one eye. This may explain some interpretive perception and response variances among normal people seeing the same object or event, depending upon which brain half receives more or less of the view. We are reminded of the aforementioned commissurotomy patient and of just how marvelous and important it is that the two hemispheres share, communicate, and integrate their experience.

## Olfactory Nerves

The olfactory nerves are not wired in crossover fashion to opposite sides of the brain. Other than some ancillary "looping" of nasal nerves to opposite brain sides, and other avenues of reciprocal communication, our nostril wiring and sense of smell are primarily homolateral. This is indicative of smell's more ancient evolutionary origins. Homolateral brain functions and nerve response mechanisms are more typical in primitive organisms or lower species. Same-side, homolateral wiring is why a lizard moves or runs the way it does, the front and rear of each side of the body moving in unison, alternating forward motion. To illustrate:

Stand up and walk by advancing your left leg and left arm together, then your right leg and right arm, and so forth. It's awkward because it works contrary to your heterolateral cerebrospinal system. Try running that way. You won't be able to. Now, walk and then run normally to see the difference and also to restore your normal heterolateral hemispheric brain-wave pattern. If you attempt the "lizard walk" for a brief time you will become strangely fatigued, somewhat imbalanced, or nervously disturbed. That's not because the homolateral movement is merely different or unfamiliar; it's because it disrupts your CNS and your eletromagnetic, etheric field. Although you may perform certain homolateral movements and even incorporate homolateral features in your body, you are predominantly a heterolaterally designed organism.

## The Nostril Cycle

The nose channels preheated, filtered air into the lungs according to a multipurpose "nostril cycle" that directs air flow alternately through each nostril. The nostril cycle is functionally established at seven months of age. Its rhythmic activity promotes an equilibrium pattern by alternating inhaled stimuli to the brain hemispheres and ensuring proper distribution of pranic (etheric) energy taken in with each breath. For smell, it reduces olfactory receptor fatigue. As with the brain hemispheres and the limbs, smell displays a dominant nostril. Many people tend to have a dominant eye, even a dominant ear as well. For most, the left ear is better than the right at recognizing melodies. Yet, for trained musicians the reverse is true. This suggests that people are more receptive and responsive to odorant stimuli received in that brain hemisphere on the same side as the dominant nostril, because the nose is homolaterally wired. Apparently, nasal blood vessels change size every few hours, alternately allowing each nasal passage to open wider than the other. Although the nostril cycle is an autonomic activity (you are not usually cognitive or consciously aware of which nostril is drawing more breath at any given time), it is possible for a person to effect the cycle subconsciously (i.e., psychosomatically) as we do so many other physiological processes, or deliberately by learned meditative breathing techniques, or even by mechanically or manually closing one nostril to invite inhaled odorant stimuli to a specific brain hemisphere, to derive a specific effect. Of course, the smell perception is communicated to the other hemisphere, but the initial, repeated, or prolonged stimuli effects register first and presumably foremost in the targeted hemisphere. (Why you would do this depends on your objectives.) Theoretically, since most people are consistently "right-sided" and therefore presumably "right-nostril dominant," their greater sensitivity and response to odors resides in the right brain—the inarticulate center of emotional feelings and aesthetic imagination. Because the hemispheres are different, scent impulses arriving through the right nostril are effectively processed differently from those arriving through the left.

The physiological response sequence—from the nose through the olfactory system, limbic system, and hypothalamus to the right hemisphere—has a psychological parallel. An instinctive sense, smell directly stimulates respondent instinctive and basic emotional urges and drives while evoking passionate and aesthetic desires, emotional memories, and imaginative concepts. Throughout the entire sequential process, the fundamental dichotomous principle of attraction/repulsion—underlying the basic either/or choices of safety/danger, like/dislike, pursuit/avoidance, acceptance/rejection—is maintained. While embellished and personalized by the more complex overtones of aesthetic evaluation and emotional feeling, the entire process, considered in isolation, is essentially subconscious, irrational, and subjective. The process activates functions of awareness (physical sensation and emotional feelings) and serves practical/physical and emotional/aesthetic motivational needs.

## The Human Mind

Yet, while the psycho-physiological process may be represented in isolation, in human beings it does not operate in isolation. As observed, odors are not strictly physical stimuli; olfaction cannot be appraised solely for the physiological effects without assessment of the emotional repercussions of odor perception. Also, the combined psycho-physiological experience cannot adequately be described by the subjective, subconscious, irrational psyche (the right brain), which is an emotionally involved, inarticulate participant in the process. Any qualitative explanation of the psycho-physiological features of the process comes from the objective, conscious, rational mind. The cognitive mind provides the logic in psychology and is the highest qualifying arbiter in psycho-physiological (psychosomatic) processes. Although the basic operation of instinctive and emotional functions of awareness and motivational needs endure in older, more original primal structures of the brain, in human beings they acquire new meaning and behavioral responses, owing to newer or more complex structural features and areas of the brain. The left hemisphere is one such structural feature—the largest cerebral repository of that component of human consciousness we term *mind.*

Providing the judiciary power of reason and the functional awareness of thought, mind is a uniquely human attribute. Indeed, *mind* is synonymous with *man.* The word *man* derives from the Indo-European root of the Sanskrit prefix *man-,* meaning "to think," and also from the Latin *mens,* "mind," and the Greek *menos,* "mind-spirit." Mind is the latest development of human consciousness. Human consciousness is the whole of our perception, functions of awareness, senses, and being, which is greater than the sum of its parts. Mind engenders the mental, intellectual motivational needs for knowledge and understanding. Ideally, mind dispassionately observes, qualifies, or modifies the instinctive and emotional behavior of the body and psyche, including that stimulated or experienced by smell. By its powers of cognition, mind mediates the effects of odors, odor perception, and odor response.

## The Mind and the Psyche

Just how much and often the mind can mediate the physical and emotional behavioral responses of smell to odors is highly problematical. At first, judged solely upon the human aptitude to identify, describe, or evaluate aromas, fragrances, and scents, the mind's involvement appears minimal. While quite capable of detecting and distinguishing odors, human beings are quite inarticulate when it comes to descriptively identifying them. As we learned earlier, there is virtually no objective language for the experience of scent. Because the evaluation of a scent—indeed, the entire process of olfactory response—is internalized and subjective, the human vocabulary for odors is limited. Odor recognition predominantly resides in the right hemisphere and therefore is largely independent of left-brain analysis, verbal memory, and speech. The left brain is somewhat "out of the loop," or outside the process. The human experience of scent is inherently the province of the psyche represented by the right brain, wherein reside the passionate, romantic, and aesthetic feelings and desires. A powerful component of the total human consciousness, the psyche is the realm of emotion and imagination. Together, psyche and mind, via the brain hemispheres, dominate human consciousness, providing the central functions of human awareness—feeling and thought—just as they share the cerebrum of the brain. Each evaluates objects and events: the one, emotionally and subjectively, the other, mentally and objectively.

## Mental Mediation

It is often said that smell is involuntary, which means that unlike closing your mouth or eyes, you cannot close your nose other than manually or mechanically, but then not for long or not without adverse consequences. One can, of course, deliberately choose to smell something, which is one way the mind can mediate the process. Nonetheless, olfaction is largely automatic. The nose is an open door through which odorants drift or are drawn whether or not we consciously wish it or even perceive them. Although it cannot deny their psycho-physiological effects, mind can in many instances anticipate odors, associatively identifying their source and providing expectations.

Perhaps most importantly, mind can anticipate, modify, restrain, or encourage the overt instinctual and emotional behavioral responses to an odorant, just as it does other psychosomatic behaviors. The left brain's detachment from odor-olfactory processing may hinder our verbal expression of the sensate, emotional experience of scents, aromas, and fragrances, but not the experience itself. Moreover, the left brain's situation is necessary to maintain mental objectivity, unclouded judgement, and reason. Lacking those qualities of mind, we would become more confined experientially, more vulnerable, and more easily persuaded.

## COGNITION AND SMELL

In terms of smell perception, cognition is more simply defined as the conscious recognition or awareness of an odor, usually bringing with that cognition associative emotional feelings, memories, and certain expectations.

An example of this comes from research at the Monell Chemical Senses Center laboratory showing that lemon oil significantly improves human perception of health and well-being. One conclusion might be that the registered responses result merely from the cognitive association of lemon scent with man-made products connoting "freshness" and "cleanliness," or with natural citrus and lemon products, like lemonade, which have the refreshingly healthy implications of summertime and outdoor activity. But such a conclusion would miss the point. First, although mediating cognitive expectations are indeed involved with the perception of odors, that alone does not disprove or preclude the genuine corresponding or independent physiologic effects of odors. It may be that cognitive expectations are justified by learned associations, acquired by personal experience, or are even genetically codified in the collective memory of the human species. In the case of lemon oil, perception is reality. We know that lemons and lemon oil are healthful and that lemon oil is psychologically uplifting and refreshing. Unless you have a peculiar genetic incompatibility or acquired emotional aversion to lemon oil (associating lemon scent to some unpleasant or traumatic event), you will expect that lemon improves health and well-being because it does. Experiments by Gerd Kobal at the University of Erlangen show that our hedonic (pleasurable) response to vanillin, the odoriferous constituent of vanilla, has little to do with cognition. Other similar experiments confirm that odors, aromas, fragrances, and scents have certain effects whether we expect them or not.

Susan Knasko, an environmental psychologist at Monell, says the idea that "good smells" are healthy and "bad smells" are not still persists at some level of the unconscious. Indeed, it does, at least in a genetic way based upon instinctive knowledge and human experience. But it also persists in the emotional subconscious, wherein like/dislike responses to an odor take on new hedonic dimensions and become more personalized. Yet, while instincts are fixed and difficult if not impossible to override, emotional feelings can be quite transient and human emotional nature highly susceptible to certain kinds of persuasion. In one experiment, Knasko placed experimental subjects in an odorless room and asked them to list any symptoms of ill-health they might have. After she told them there was an "unpleasant" odor in the room, although there wasn't, they listed even more symptoms. An imagined malodor had made them feel less healthy. Knasko's experiment tells us a great deal about the influence of suggestion and of outside opinion upon the irrational emotional nature. Besides suggestion, the countless origins and combinations of real cognitive factors (memories, learned or acquired behaviors and responses, and temporary moods) that are inextricably linked to odors make scientific analysis of an odorant's actual effects more complicated. Yet, while the mediating effects of cognitive factors may hamper or obscure olfactory research, they do not diminish or prevent it.

## The Subliminal Influence of Odors

The involuntary nature of smell permits access and response to unperceived odorants as well as to detectable odors. Odors introduced below the smell perception or detection threshold can nonetheless produce psycho-physiological responses. You needn't be consciously aware of an odor for it to effect psycho-physiological changes and influence your behavior. As demonstrated by Tyler Lorig of the psychology department at Washington & Lee University in Virginia, not all odor effects involve cognition. In his experiment, a synthetic musk administered below detectable threshold levels, hence below cognitive awareness, produced a considerable reduction in alpha brain-wave activity resulting in poorer performance of a task requiring mental concentration. The selection of odorants is significant. Musk is a sexually stimulating pheromonal-like substance hardly conducive to tasks of mental concentration. Predictably, it proved distracting, but more so because it was subliminally, rather than cognitively, introduced. The mind can mediate in the olfaction process if it is cognizant of the odor by smell perception or has other knowledge of the odor's presence. Your nose may initially recoil at the smell of garlic, but the mind, reason, can persuade you to try it at least once or often enough that you accept or even come to enjoy garlic. The mind can dissuade you from ingesting a liquid that smells good but isn't. In each instance, the mind has knowledge (that garlic is healthful, that the sweet liquid is poison) not possessed by your senses or feelings. Mind gains that cognitive knowledge by means other than simpler cognition based upon olfactory awareness. Carbon monoxide—an odorless, colorless, and deadly gas—will not arouse olfaction, but your reason will tell you to avoid it by knowledge of its sources and likely presence.

## Odors and Sleep Modification

In no other situation is the involuntary nature of smell more evident than in the state of sleep. Peter Badia, a Bowling Green State University professor, is learning that even when you are asleep, your nose is awake, albeit somewhat drowsily. People are responsive to odors much as they are to other sensory stimuli introduced into their sleep (e.g., sound, light). That is, their response is not all that alert unless a stimulus is strong enough to awaken them. Like responses from other senses, olfaction responses greatly diminish in sleep for the same reasons: so you will get your rest and because in sleep your consciousness recedes into unconsciousness, which then runs on "auto-pilot." Other than Professor Badia's work, little research has been done on sleep and smell. Conversely, there is plenty of research indicating the effects of odors in waking states, psychological and physiological, using equipment to measure brain waves, heart rate, and other bodily functions. Badia wanted to see whether certain fragrances deemed relaxing or alerting in waking states would function likewise in sleep. Students tested in the university sleep lab, by both objective and subjective lab equipment techniques (monitors for heart rate, brain-wave activity, respiration, and muscle tension as well as later respondent questionnaires about the quality of their sleep) were randomly exposed to either normal room air or a specific fragrance. All measured analyses showed that sleepers reacted more strongly to the odor than to normal air. But in virtually all cases, regardless of its relaxing or alerting attribution, the fragrance disrupted sleep. By disrupting sleep, peppermint, an alerting substance, performed as expected. Owing to its presumed relaxing effects, jasmine was expected to enhance sleep but instead proved disrupting. Thought to be relaxing, coumarin, a common plant extract component found in some essential oils and used as a fixative in cosmetics, toiletries, and tobacco, was also disruptive. Once again, as in the Tyler Lorig experiment using synthetic musk oil, the selection of fragrances is significant.

First, it is uncertain whether certain fragrances used were complete essential oils or synthetic or otherwise incomplete extracts. Badia selected scents based upon earlier lab findings and those selected by his sponsor, the Fragrance Foundation (FF), an international fragrance industry group that through its Fragrance Research Fund (FRF) subsidizes research into the effects of perfume upon human behavior. Badia's peppermint was, in fact, pepperine, not the essential oil. Second, the assumption of jasmine's relaxing effects is somewhat mistaken. Jasmine (the essential oil, anyway) is normalizing and more often has an arousing effect, as Japanese studies have shown. Professor Shizuo Torii and his colleagues at Toho University School of Medicine in Tokyo, showed that jasmine increases alertness by stimulating beta brain-wave activity and the CNV (contingent negative variable), both attention brainwaves, as measured by EEG (electroencephalogram) or CNV amplitude. Dr. Paolo Rovesti has used jasmine essential oil for depression, an aromatherapy use consistent with jasmine's characteristics as an antidepressant and euphoric. If indeed real jasmine essence was used in Badia's experiment, it performed just as it should.

Certainly coumarin, a chemical lactone component removed from a plant extract, is no essential oil. Neither is heliotropin, an aromatic aldehyde used in perfumery and otherwise to impart a sweet "almond vanilla" fragrance. (It is uncertain whether heliotropin—aka piperonal—actually occurs in vanilla beans and also whether the actual scent of the heliotrope flower is attributable to piperonal, which is used to simulate lilac, carnation, and other floral bouquet odors.) Badia observed that heliotropin was the only fragrance tested that did not disrupt sleep, showing instead a slight but statistically insignificant tendency to enhance it. Meanwhile, at the Memorial Sloan-Kettering Cancer Center in New York, research headed by William H. Redd, a Center psychologist, found in a study of eighty-five patients that those exposed to heliotropin during their MRI (magnetic resonance imaging) diagnostic procedure experienced 63 percent less anxiety than the control group patients who received the usual moistened air through the same delivery system. (The study was presented in March 1991 at the meeting of the Society of Behavioral Medicine in Washington, D.C.) Professor Redd reminds us that MRI scanning requires the patient to remain motionless for as long as ninety minutes inside a small cylinder. People routinely experience high anxiety, even claustrophobic reactions or panic attacks. Typically, 10 percent of patients quit the test before completion, regardless of the lost expense of the terminated procedure—about $1,500. The news that heliotropin dramatically induces relaxation in a waking anxiety state, while having a virtually neutral effect upon an already relaxed state of sleep, points up the stark difference between the two states of consciousness. Sleep eliminates cognitive expectations about odors and also reduces observable emotional responsive behavior. Despite later test questionnaires, people seldom accurately recount their actual sleeping mood or behavioral responses, much less their dreams. A great deal of emotionally charged activity, which might be observable in the waking state, goes on almost silently during sleep and especially in the dream state. Dream analysis is difficult, inexact, and subject to interpretation. Professor Badia concludes that current evidence strongly suggests that odors disrupt sleep, but the evidence suggesting whether odors can enhance sleep is weak. Yet, how much of the recorded agitation of the tested sleepers was owing to or compounded by coincidental but forgotten sleep and dream activity? Can an odorant's effects be assessed by dream behavior, events, and feelings? Since sleep is the quintessential relaxed state, how much more relaxed can it really be made by odorants? Probably not much.

Smell is a reflexive sense; olfaction does not, cannot, unilaterally decide to selectively ignore a registerable odor. Like hearing, smell is a constant sleep alarm for protection. Also like hearing, smell reacts less discriminately to stimuli during sleep than it does during waking, thereby more readily causing arousal. Quite naturally, sleep disturbance is to be expected from odors or sounds, especially intrusive ones—in which case, the results of Badia's research raise possibilities for the use of odors to arouse comatose patients. The logic of treating an unconscious state (coma) by the subconscious sense of smell, rather than, say, electroconvulsive shock, may offer distinct advantages.

Aromatherapy makes no claims for synthetic fragrances, incomplete extracts, or isolated components. The demonstrable somnifacient (soporific) and sedative characteristics of authentic essential oils have a natural, intelligently homeostatic affect upon sleep: they induce and enhance it. Yet, the quality of sleep itself is a variable estimation. For example, insomniacs are often heard to say that they never sleep, or couldn't fall asleep last night, or sleep too little and/or very badly. Yet, sleep observation studies prove just as often that those same "insomniacs" do indeed sleep—longer, more often, and better than they say or believe. Genuine, chronic, severe insomnia (sleep deprivation) is a real but rare condition, usually associated with mental illness. Most types of insomnia are mild, transient, exaggerated, or quite imaginary. (Some insomniacs actually dream that they don't sleep.) You can easily give yourself the suggestion to awaken at a certain time without an alarm clock or awaken in the night at the faintest cry of your newborn infant or sick child. In Badia's study, what effect did his preliminary instructions to the sleep participants—which were to awaken or attempt to awaken if they detected an odor—have upon their responses? In fact, whether the participants actually awakened or only stirred (they did both), they recorded sleep disturbance. Did his wake-up suggestion further condition their arousal, heightening their anticipation and responses to the randomly introduced odors? It seems we have as much to learn about sleep olfaction as we do about sleep itself. Observations and study of the certain sleep and subliminal effects of odors have, however, resolved our own version of the rather self-centered phenomenological question ("If a tree falls in the forest and no one is there to hear it fall, does it make any sound?"): If we can't smell it, does it still affect us? Be assured, the answer to both questions is yes.

## The Influence of Odors Upon the Mind

We ought to be at least as concerned about how odors affect cognition as we are about how cognition mediates the effects of odors. Since odors act more directly upon the instinctual and emotional areas and structures of the brain (limbic system, hypothalamus, right brain) and less directly upon the mind (left brain), we ought not to be surprised that odor-induced feelings (like otherwise generated feelings) influence thought content and the thinking process, mental concentration, and perhaps even rational judgement. Psychologically, moods are complex, transient, largely emotional states assembled from dichotomous (good/bad) feelings, past and current cognitive evaluations and associations (of circumstances, conditions, and events), and biological, physiological states and processes. In most people, moods strongly affect or largely determine every behavior from eating habits to social conduct.

Howard Ehrlichman, of the City University of New York Psychology Department, has reported on an experiment that showed how pleasant and unpleasant odors affect performance in a basic creativity task: predictably, when smelling a pleasant odor, students performed decidedly better. In other experimental research financially supported by the Fragrance Research Fund (FRF), the team of Ehrlichman and J. N. Halpern, while attempting to minimize cognitive association, employed "pleasant" and "unpleasant" odors to induce positive or negative emotional states or moods. Unsurprisingly, and as happens with other normally occurring or deliberately induced moods (invariably patterned along dichotomous emotional evaluations—pleasurable/unpleasurable, happy/unhappy, etc.), the odors directed personal memories toward typically similar hedonic reflections. Subjects inhaling a pleasant odor recalled happier memories than those recalled by subjects who inhaled unpleasant odors.

From another experiment funded by the FRF, the laboratory condition observations of Ehrlichman and Linda Bastone suggest that unpleasant odors have a more profound impression on moods than do pleasant odors. This can in no way be considered conclusive, however, because the results are largely dependent upon a person's preexisting mood when the odor is administered. If you are already in a positive mood, a pleasant odor will not enhance that positivity as dramatically as an unpleasant odor will detract from it. Conversely, if you are already in an emotionally negative state, a pleasant odor will more dramatically elevate your mood than an unpleasant odor is likely to worsen it. Although a given odor can measurably improve a negative mood or undermine a positive one, there are limits to how strong that effect will be, largely depending upon the person, the situation or circumstances, and the nature and strength of the odorant. Logically, the limits of an odorant to further enhance or exacerbate a preexisting positive or negative mood become narrower still. Therefore, the comparative effectiveness of unpleasant or pleasant odors becomes highly debatable in the opposing attitudinal approaches of aversion therapy versus positive reinforcement, whereby the relative merits of reward and punishment (pleasure or displeasure) are, in that context, dramatized by using odors to condition or modify human behavior.

## Brain Chemistry

Some of the altering effects that odors have upon mood may be caused by their alteration of endogenous brain opioids: suppressing them (unpleasant odors) or accelerating them (pleasant odors). These endogenous (originating or produced from within) opiates have narcotic-like effects. We know that the antidepressant, sedative effects of essential oils are partly attributable to their consequential release of endorphins and enkephalins—neurochemical analgesics and tranquilizers. In this regard, however, the effects of a simple chemical odorant, having far fewer and less complex or intelligent properties and characteristics than does an essential oil, ought not to be overestimated or thought comparable. Nonetheless, the release of naturally occurring brain chemicals is quite possibly how an unpleasant experience, such as MRI screening, is mitigated by a pleasant odor like heliotropin. The cognitive associative factors must be considered too, since fond memories of a pleasant odor will likewise trigger endogenous releases. For example, a pleasant odor that has pleasurable associative meaning to a person will further increase endogenous opiate levels in the brain beyond those created by an otherwise pleasant but less meaningful scent. This becomes tricky because of the unknown associative variables involving scents and personal memory. Not only must the odorant's nature and properties be considered (all odors are not created equal), but the administering of it could be counterproductive.

Despite many common assumptions about odors, defining a "pleasant" odor is still largely a personal and always subjective evaluation. Obviously, the administering of an expectedly pleasant odor that nonetheless has uniquely unpleasant personal connotations would only make the situation worse owing to resistance to the odor. The intrinsic value of the aromatic substance or odorant used, and the associated meaning or connotation it might have to a given person, are two important considerations for effective, individualized treatment in any proposed therapy or experiment involving scents, fragrances, or aromas. Owing to the pliability of some emotional associations, it is possible to teach or condition a person to enjoy a previously disliked or less significant odor. Clinically speaking, there may be reason to do so: to overcome a psychological block or aversion, or to create a new cognitive experience without past associations by reassociation with a new, positive experience. Otherwise, behavioral techniques that attempt to teach a patient to associate a familiar, commonly accepted odor (e.g., chocolate, as is used by Dr. Susan Schiffman, or apricot) with a state of relaxation are generally more successful because the patient is less resistant; but they are nevertheless bound by the nature and product quality of the scent substance used. Such techniques involve scent as a psychological device rather than as a therapeutic agent. Therefore, the existent or nonexistent virtues of the aromatic substance are incidental and are usually considered irrelevant by the psychotherapist so long as the patient finds it otherwise pleasant and does not reject it. It is the relaxation technique that matters; the odor is only a cue. At Syracuse University, assistant professor of psychology Michael Carey has exposed cancer patients to positively associated odors to mitigate the negative associations to chemotherapy. Because chemotherapy is so painfully unpleasant, some patients begin experiencing nausea—even vomiting—merely in expectation of it. By using rose scent, Carey attempts to comfort the patients.

While praiseworthy for their motives, these and similar clinical applications of scent to modify behavior are not authentic aromatherapy. Regarding scent selection, even assuming that the cancer patients received true rose otto—highly unlikely for many reasons—rose would not be among an aromatherapist's first choices for the situation. Needless to say, there are no essential oils of apricot or chocolate. What takes place, in the instance of relaxation techniques especially, is simple Pavlovian-style conditioning.

In the chemotherapy example, as happened in the MRI experiment using heliotropin, the basic element of distraction is operative in the response. Ironically, even if Professor Carey's intention was that rose scent could later be used to remind patients of their calm feelings, because of the same conditioning responsible for the relaxation responses to apricot or chocolate it might only be a matter of time before the cancer patients begin to negatively associate rose scent with the entire unpleasantness of chemotherapy.

Pure, natural, complete essential oils are superior to other odorous or aromatic substances. But regardless of whether real essential oils are used in behavioral techniques, true aromatherapy does not rely upon psychological conditioning to be effective, although positive association can certainly be made and ordinarily is part of an aromatherapy experience (e.g., aromatherapy massage). Aromatherapy relies upon the actual properties and characteristics of essential oils, which are active, independently therapeutic agents, not placebos. Neither are essential oils merely scented cues or distractions. Unlike synthetics and isolated chemical constituents, essential oils do not artificially exploit olfaction to create superficial or temporary effects, and they are not merely olfactory stimuli. Essential oils convey healthful information to the body and brain, and because they have genuine, natural therapeutic benefits, the nonhabituating effects of essential oils do not decline by repeated application. Neither will they exhaust the brain or body's responses. In fact, they safely strengthen them.

## Odors and Performance

Sponsored by the Fragrance Foundation, two University of Cincinnati psychology professors, William N. Dember and Joel Warm, tested the effects of certain odors upon human performance. Their study findings, "The Effects of Odor on Performance and Stress" presented in February 1991 at the annual meeting of the American Association for the Advancement of Science, concluded that scents are able to sustain alertness and improve performance in routine tasks. Some subjects, while engaged in a forty-minute vigilance test requiring them to press a button whenever a certain line pattern appeared on a video screen, were occasionally given a brief burst of peppermint or muguet (lily of the valley) scent through an oxygen mask. Others were supplied whiffs of plain air. According to Dember, the performance of those participants who breathed the two odors was as much as 25 percent more accurate than that of the plain-air group. (A replication study at the Catholic University Psychology Department by Raja Parasuraman, another FRF grant recipient, produced the same results by using only peppermint. Once again, an industry group, International Flavors and Fragrances, selected the scent.) In his conclusion that fragrances can affect mood, Professor Dember subscribes to the idea that scents activate specific chemical "brain messengers" or neurotransmitters.

In these instances, pleasant scents positively affected the participants' moods, modifying behavior toward a better performance—at least in a routine task. We cannot attest to the authenticity of the scents employed in the experiments. Considering the sponsor, we suspect synthetics again were used. There is no distilled essential oil of lily of the valley (muguet). Although we are told that a satisfactory concréte has been developed using butane as the solvent, the natural flower oil is not a commercial item, owing to natural production limitations and the prevalence of perfume-grade muguet scent reproduced by blending synthetic ingredients and natural isolated chemical components. Cognition certainly played a role in the studies by Dember and Warm and by Parasuraman. Unlike the Lorig experiment, which introduced a distracting scent (synthetic musk) at subliminal levels that undermined mental concentration, these two tests overtly presented a mentally stimulating fragrance (peppermint or pepperine), which correctly translated into increased performance.

## Odors and Judgement

We have already explained how the mind can mediate in the olfaction process if it is cognizant of the odor or has other knowledge of the odor's presence. The mind can also mediate an odor experience by modifying the mood or the resultant behavior despite having no knowledge at all of the odor. It does this the same way it modifies any behavior (by self-control or mental discipline) but only if the mind is self-consciously aware of the behavior or the mood and then seeks to change it in any way by conscious effort. It is worth repeating that functionally, the left brain's more remote situation from the olfactory process is necessarily important to maintain mental poise and objectivity, unclouded judgement, and reason, preventing the mind from becoming unduly influenced by odors— i.e., more easily persuaded by or made vulnerable to the changes of mood or emotional status instigated or altered by odors (or for that matter any other emotionally appealing stimuli). Ideally, the developed mind (left brain) prevents man from "losing his head" in emotional situations or otherwise acting irrationally. In this context, to whatever greater degree the mind is cognitively engaged in the smell process, or where odors intrude into more vital, serious mental processes, to that degree the mind will mediate the effects of odors, and those effects will proportionately decline in influence, unless consciously sanctioned and permitted by the mind. It could be said that the left brain operates consciously to forestall "mind-control" by odors and submission to their emotional effects—again, provided that at some point the mind is cognitively aware of the odor by smell perception, or has reasoned knowledge of the odor's subliminal presence, or is attentive to any mood or behavioral changes caused by that odor. At that time, the mind must arbitratively decide whether to allow, resist, or otherwise interventionally modify the process.

Olfactory research into the effects of odors on cognition confirms the mind's important role in the process. Whereas odors may be considered functionally equivalent to emotional mood in their effects upon less consciously controlled cognitive processes (e.g., those involved in personal creativity, memory, recall, or simpler mental tasks), odors are not by themselves operationally influential in more consciously controlled cognitive judgements—i.e., at higher levels of cognition when conscious reasoning and rational evaluations are involved. In the aforementioned studies by Ehrlichman and Bastone, testing the effects of pleasant or unpleasant odors upon mood and performance, the creativity of the pleasant-odor group was significantly higher than that of the unpleasant-odor group (a no-odor, plain-air group scored in between). But no such significant differences were observed among the three odor groups during considered scenarios that presented to the participants perceived risks and involving assistance to others. While showing that odors have effects that parallel moods—that is, produced feeling states that function similarly to moods—the more conscious, rational mental processes involved in evaluating risks, thinking situations, and so on were unaffected by scent.

Another phase of the Ehrlichman and Bastone experiments found significantly more positive ratings in people's judgements of slide pictures of human faces and of word meaning associations when participants breathed pleasant odors instead of unpleasant odors. Once again, we see how elements of mood can transform objective reasoning. But it should be noted that typically, as is the case here, these judgements are not particularly or profoundly crucial or critical. Moreover, the differences were apparent only among respondents found to be highly "field dependent"—that is, people whose judgement is strongly influenced by environmental factors.

Such results might invite conclusions that no odor can directly affect serious rational judgement, concentration, or other mental processes, either positively or negatively. We have discussed throughout how the strong and healthy mind should ideally function; but in reality, the powers of mind do not always prevail. People remain largely irrational and emotional. Moods, and presumably therefore whatever might contribute to those moods, can indeed influence rational judgements. Often, in many people, the mind—reason, intellect, thought—is lax, undisciplined, unobservant, inattentive, lacking intellectual discrimination and concentration, easily distracted and submerged by emotional feelings, or overruled by habit, instinctive reflexive behavior, or environmental factors. As is true of odors, not all minds or brains are created equal.

Consider, too, that the mind more often mediates the effects of odors communicating to the left brain indirectly—e.g., across the corpus callosum from the right brain, which more eagerly receives smell input. But are odors homolaterally transmitted to the left brain via the left nostril and olfactory nerve mediated any differently? Are their effects stronger owing to more direct homolateral association or sympathy, or are they instead even weaker owing to the more "head-on" encounter with the less susceptible half of the brain? The answers to these questions depend somewhat upon the status of each person's mind and upon the nature and strength of the odor introduced.

Olfaction remains predominantly a right brain phenomenon. Generally speaking, owing to its own highly developed neural complexity, the left brain assents only to the most complex, intelligent odors. In the research test just described, as in others, synthetic scents or single isolated aromatic components were used. (Ehrlichman and Bastone used almond extract and muguet as pleasant odors; the sulfurous and rancid odors of thiophene and butyric acid as unpleasant scents.) These may be adequate to the task of mere stimulation—eliciting basic biochemical responses from older, more primitive areas and structures of the brain (e.g., the limbic and olfactory systems and the hypothalamus), prompting simple recall, and effecting mood changes or memory and emotional hedonic responses via the right brain but without having much impression on the left brain hemisphere, directly or otherwise.

In every way, the use of superior aromatic substances will evoke superior responses in all of the appropriate organs and areas of the brain. In the left brain particularly, only superior aromatics will do. Essential oils are just such substances, complex and intelligent enough to communicate with the left brain directly. Here, too, such possibilities depend upon the character of the given oil itself. Not just complex, it must also have a natural specific affinity for the mind and the left brain thought processes. Unlike simple perfumes, fragrances, and aromas, essential oils have the best and highest communicative and evocative potential upon both brain hemispheres. If the left brain can be specifically affected by an odor, that odor will have to be one worthy of the mind.

## Moods: Emotion and the Development of Olfaction

The development of our olfactory sense and use of scent follows our physical, emotional, mental, and social evolution. A more advanced, complex organism makes more advanced, complex uses of its existing senses. Likewise, it also evolves and develops senses with accompanying physical and psychological features and structures to meet the more advanced, complex needs of its progressive development. In human beings, sight, hearing, and language have superseded smell and scent as means of distant and social communication, of awareness and perception, and of gaining and transferring knowledge. This is not only because man's sense of smell has somewhat atrophied or become less capable today than it was in prehistoric times—or, for that matter, before humans walked upright—but also because sight, hearing, and verbal communication are more efficient, important, and valuable to our more complex environment and expanding consciousness. Although certainly our existing sense of smell can be trained to improve (e.g., to overcome smell disorders or heighten aesthetic appreciation), it will never regain its lost preeminence and significance, at least not as it once was or as it still is among other animals. This is a consequence of expanding, advancing consciousness; and human consciousness is the most advanced, varied, and complex of all animal species. Expanding, evolving consciousness requires and creates expanded, improved sensory apparatus and appreciations and psychological functions of awareness.

Today, scent and smell (and taste) as means of aesthetic expression and socialization, rather than as tools for survival, are more of a luxury than a necessity. Brought out of the plain world of natural reality and physical survival into the imaginative realms of romance and erotic fantasy, smell is more aesthetically and less instinctively utilized to improve the quality of existence rather than the chances of survival. We compensate our rudimentary power of smell with saturation—a veritable glut of odors, scents, fragrances, and aromas. The food and fragrance industries exploit and capitalize on this marvelous change in our sense of smell by providing us with a plethora of scents, fragrances, and aromas designed to titillate and amuse our sense of smell, arouse our emotions, adjust our moods, and express our feelings.

America's first great psychologist, William James, credited the human organism with having a larger number of instincts than any of the lower animals—a reasonable supposition, since instinct is a biological and physiological function, and the human being is the most complex biophysiological unit on earth. What distinguishes *Homo sapiens* from the rest of the animal kingdom is not that we have shed our animal nature but that we have added to it mind and higher emotional feelings, which in turn may mask our instincts and alter our biological emotions but have not erased them. Instincts are our oldest habits—the things we learned so well in our forgotten past (involving all the fundamental activities of survival and existence) that we can do them literally in our sleep, autonomically, without thinking. Next to them are natural biological emotions, the more primitive "gut-feelings" originating from our bodies and, mixed with instinct, linked to physical processes, functions of awareness (sensation), and the body's physical/practical motivational needs. Above the biological emotions are uniquely human emotions not held by other animals: a wider spectrum of secondary, learned, or acquired feelings ranging from the heavenly to the hideous, also tied to our body responses (whereby they affect us psychosomatically) but originating in our more complex psychological processes.

Sometimes human emotions color, mingle, or correspond with biological emotions, turning natural anger into cruelty or hatred, simple fear into complexes or phobias, or transforming biological emotional needs for security, protection, physical closeness, and comfort into human emotional desires for companionship, attention and affection. The biological emotions function more through the primitive brain areas of the limbic system and hypothalamus, whereas both the lower and the higher human emotions are centered in the right hemisphere of the brain. We often describe our lower human emotions—not just our biological emotions—as "animal behavior," but this is a misapprehension and an injustice to other animals. Animal biological emotions may be common and crude, but they are also innocent and natural. Our self-conscious lower emotions—hate, jealousy, envy, and the rest—are as uniquely human as our higher feelings of sympathy, compassion, and tenderness.

Human emotions lend an amazing texture to human experience, thought, and consciousness. We possess passions, desires, and sensibilities of the psyche neither enjoyed nor suffered by other animals. As a unique quality of human consciousness, the psyche provides us the functional awareness of feelings, emotional/aesthetic motivational needs, and the power of imagination. Our emotional nature (our feelings and desires) operates along the dichotomous principle of attraction/repulsion. Sometimes strongly passionate and always subjective, our personal desires and emotional evaluations (like/dislike) are not always in our own or others' best interests. Often we discover that just because something "feels good" or "feels right" doesn't necessarily mean it is good or is right. One can be made to feel confidently justified about many erroneous things. There is a delusional quality to emotion that accompanies the gift of imagination. Alternately, feelings are easily manipulated and persuaded or resistantly biased and opinionated. The devotional, irrational qualities of emotion lead us into blind belief. Swayed by appearances and circumstances, amenable to suggestion, we often mistake our feelings for reality, attributing them to the wrong source or stimuli, which may be environmental or social factors or may have personally generated psycho-physiological origins.

Emotion is affected by various outside stimuli and subjective impressions. Although frequently unreliable, transitory, and readily spent, feelings are better kept soft and malleable to enable us to form temporary opinions about inner and outer reality, about which we ought not to draw hasty conclusions based solely upon emotion. Persistent negative emotions, and "hard feelings" bind us to prejudices, irrational superstitions, fears, phobias, obsessions, compulsions, habits, and a host of psychosomatic illnesses wired into corresponding areas of the brain and adopted by the musculature, posture, and responses of the body. Contrastingly, healthy emotions and positive feelings are a special source of pleasure and enjoyment that enriches our experience. But the frequent or excessive indulgence of emotion, positive or negative, has a disturbing effect upon homeostasis and psychological balance.

The evaluative criterion of emotion is acceptance/rejection, about which we may be reflexively passive or reactionary. The mind is necessary to restore balance to this seesaw activity of emotions. Because it is inherently reflective, our emotional nature lacks the prospective capacity given to the mind—the ability to project beyond past or present circumstances. Emotion is for the moment; unlike mind, it does not plan ahead or consider consequences outside its own immediate interests. By thought and reason we are able to analyze, correlate, and organize our experiential information; to grasp analogy and by speculation and theory to expand our consciousness, learning, knowledge, and communication. We become capable of making impersonal, disinterested judgements based upon objective criteria other than our immediate, self-absorbed emotional desires and concerns. Moreover, as it advises, governs, informs, and observes our feelings and behavior, mind represents and cultivates conscience.

A strong and healthy mind strives to sustain good, positive moods such as optimism and elation and to dispel bad, negative moods such as despair and pessimism while maintaining a psychological serenity—a clear, calm sea of emotions. Unless otherwise wrapped in emotional feelings, thoughts and ideas are inherently neutral—i.e., unemotional—but the exchange between mood and mind is reciprocal, and often their conditions are shared, good or bad thoughts accompanying good or bad feelings accordingly. A later evolutionary development than the psyche, mind has yet to gain complete ascendancy in human consciousness. At least as often as not, emotion manages to submerge reason, blur intuition, and distort instinct—the latter two being separate judiciary powers or perceptive functions of awareness, with which feelings are often confused. It is symptomatic of our lack of discriminate understanding in irrational or unconscious matters of human behavior that we often reveal this confusion by using the three terms—instinct, intuition, feeling—interchangeably. Otherwise, the equilibrated integration of good thoughts and good feelings produces cognitive assonance—a consistency of response and behavior that denotes self-control.

Our understanding of human emotional nature provides insight into our use of smell. As mankind evolved, our feelings and our sense of smell developed coextensively beyond the function that smell and biological feelings mutually serve in animals. Animals have instincts and basic pleasurable biological feelings without the best or worst connotations ascribed to human feelings. In the rest of the animal kingdom, instinct still rules; animals have no personal desires or passions, and their feelings and instincts, like their sense of smell, serve the perpetuation of their species. Only human beings are emotionally introspective, using feelings to define themselves and their personal experience; to this purpose smell has now been enlisted.

Animals make no such subjective psychological or aesthetic uses of smell and scents. For animals, smell and scent are strictly biological matters of practical importance. Their olfactory sense and odoriferous secretions are designed to receive and convey accurate fundamental messages among themselves, carrying necessary survival information about their natural existence and environment, such as health, sustenance, procreation, territory, and enemies. The olfaction process in animals is a more precise, specific, no-frills affair and is hence more reliable. Unlike human beings, animals are not so easily duped or deceived by scents; they have no psychological moods to contend with or "atmospheric" moods to create.

## Smell Response: Scent Preferences and Personality

Connected with the older, more primitive parts of the brain, the human senses of touch, taste, and smell—the chemical senses—were the first to evolve in man and remain the first to develop in infancy. By adding upon each sense—touch, taste, smell, sight, hearing—an organism expands its perceptive range and capacity to handle increasingly complex stimuli. As such, man has attained a visual and auditory dominance more suitable to his advanced consciousness and wider experience. Recapitulating human evolution, three-month-old babies show highly developed brain responses to food aromas, well before their visual and auditory senses similarly develop in later maturity. Although some responses to odors are clearly learned, infants as young as nine-months old already respond to pleasant or unpleasant scents by physical behaviors, such as facial expressions and body movements, much like those of adults. It is not only our emotional conditioning and learned habits, but our instinctive, reflexive responses to odors that make them so attractive or even compelling throughout life and allow our amenable smell to be favorably or unfavorably exploited. By three years of age, children have the same smell preferences as adults; although they do not as readily discriminate between "good" or "bad" odors, instead later learning more refined discriminatory behavior. Maturity increases aesthetic sophistication and individuality in scent preferences. Still closer and more responsive to their animal nature, children tend to reject complex adult perfumes and colognes, preferring instead, if at all, single-note or simpler fragrances, especially those having a floral or fruity bouquet. (Children likewise enjoy fruity flavors more than do adults.)

## Gender Differences in Olfactory Response

The differences between gender scent preferences and smell responses are also evident from infancy. Female infants are more attentive to scented artifacts than are male babies. In a Vanderbilt University study done by George Porter, female babies a mere one to three days old remained focused on a new scent for longer periods than did same-age male infants, who instead turned their heads alternately, from side to side, equally and more often when presented with new scents, spending no more time upon one scent than the other. From birth, women seem to have a greater olfactory aptitude sensitivity and response to odors than do men. Women are more able to detect odorants in lower-level concentrations and are better able to identify odors of all kinds. The first capability derives from their inborn reproductive protection skills, whereby they can better safeguard the fetus during pregnancy. The second has more to do with learning and familiarity, since females are intrinsically more interested in scents than are males.

In nearly all respects, women are generally more adept than men in matters of olfaction. But the superior performance of the female sense of smell undergoes greater fluctuations than its male counterpart, owing not only to wider hormonal changes connected with ovulation, pregnancy, and menopause but to other biological, psychological, and environmental factors as well. Just as it is from birth (the "morning" of life), female smell acuity is usually sharpest in the morning hours of the day, slowly declining as the day progresses. By contrast, male olfaction is constant throughout the day and by afternoon equals that of women, after which both peak again around midnight. It has long been observed that women are more emotionally sensitive than men—a psychological difference that has biological correspondences and a definite influence on, and correlation to, women's sense of smell. Women are more right-brain oriented and influenced than are men. Although there are varying degrees of left-brain dominance among all people, left-brain dominance is more pronounced in males than in females. More than that, there are structural gender differences in the human brain that account for corresponding differences in how the two sexes think, feel, respond, and behave.

Only within the past few years have scientists noted or delineated the significant structural difference of the corpus callosum (the fibers connecting the brain hemispheres) between men and women. Even more recently, another study, reported at the November 1990 meeting of the Society of Neuroscience, has found yet another gender-related difference in a brain feature known as the sylvian fissure. According to neuropsychologist Sandra Witelson, author of the study, "These results suggest that the female brain is not just a scaled-down version of the male brain." (A man's brain is larger and heavier than that of a woman.) "It actually has a different shape, and the same parts do different things." Summarily, the female brain, in addition to being smaller, is organized differently: the communication between the hemispheres is different, and the focus of consciousness is more right-brain than left-brain. Consequently, women respond, behave, think, and feel differently from men, which reflects in women's olfaction and scent preferences. Regarding these gender differences in brain anatomy, adds Witelson, "There must be some genetic influence for this brain morphology to develop as it does," and whatever that may be, it begins in the womb, apparently triggered by sex hormone activity.

Because in human beings scent and smell are analogous to feelings and moods, we can expect the hedonic responses, aesthetic tastes, and smell preferences of men and women to reflect, both qualitatively and quantitatively, the differences in their emotional natures. The fragrance industry has learned that men are typically attracted to complex floral and spicy fragrances, women to simple, single-note fragrances. Males seek consistency in their choices—one good, favorite cologne—whereas women change their perfumes more easily and readily. Noting women's heightened awareness and response to scents and their more capricious scent preferences, the fragrance industry directs its marketing far more toward women than men by the psychological and aesthetic allure of its products. These include not just personal perfumes but a host of scented household products and items, cosmetics and toiletries, which exploit the female emotional nature and capitalize on a woman's instinctive safety response to scents that are "clean" and "fresh." By nature, women are a more interested, hence larger and more renewable segment of the market for scented items of all kinds. It is easier and more profitable to sell scents to women than to men.

## Female Psychology

Not just more emotionally malleable, changeable, and sensitive, women are more vulnerable, susceptible, and responsive to mood changes from various causes. "Emotions are contagious," observed the famed Swiss psychoanalyst Carl Gustav Jung, and numerous scientific studies since Jung's time have confirmed the accuracy of his observation. The more recent of these studies indicate how women participate or indulge in personal and social behavior that perpetuates emotional contagion, both as transmitters and receivers of emotional signals, energies, and vibrations.

Studies done by many psychologists, such as Elaine Hatfield at the University of Hawaii and Ellen Sullins at Northern Arizona University, attest to the instantaneous, unconscious, and somewhat insidious transmission of emotions or moods. This transmission is accomplished by a subtle and complex communication and mimicry of body langauge, facial expressions, physical touch, psychic impressions (via the astral-etheric aura), odor exchanges, and talk. According to Ohio State University psychologist John Cacciopo, the more emotionally expressive people are, the more likely they are to transmit their moods to other people during conversation. Meanwhile, people who are easily affected by the moods of others have especially forceful autonomic reactions (psycho-physiological responses) to emotionally expressive people. Although men are by no means immune to emotional contagion, for biological and psychological reasons they more cautiously resist it. More eagerly willing to share and express their feelings, women more easily and more often promote emotional contagion.

Being disposed to share and express their emotions, women are more readily able to verbalize their feelings because the female corpus callosum allows easier internal cross-talk between the brain hemispheres. The female corpus callosum provides a less resistant, but also less discriminatory, demarcation inclined to commingle or blur the distinction between the activities and roles of the brain hemispheres. This is why women, along with their readiness to express feelings, are more apt to verbally describe odors and articulate their mood-altering effects. Men are more apt to employ language for the communication of ideas and to exchange objective information and knowledge, rather than express subjective emotions or impressions, which may have personal significance but less practical or socially transferable value and usefulness. The frequent female complaint that men will not or cannot share or express their feelings arises from the real brain differences between the sexes and the relative value and emphasis each places upon emotional transmission. Like tuning forks vibrating at the same pitch, a feeling of sympathetic unity or symbiosis occurs between people as they synchronize their moods, which is something women seek to achieve and do more often among themselves. But the more emotionally motivated nature of women, and their greater tendency for internal dialogue and external verbalization of feelings, has its advantages and disadvantages. More sympathetic and inclined to commiseration, women are more susceptible to emotional contagion of all kinds. Observational studies of people's moods show that while saying they are as happy as men, women report being in negative moods twice as often as males and retain negative moods for longer periods of time. According to psychologist Ed Diener at the University of Illinois, "One reason seems to be that women's moods tend to be more intense than men's." In short, they have higher peaks and lower valleys, and more of them.

The higher reported number of negative moods and the greater mood fluctuations among women are consequences of the emotionally centered female nature, greater exposure to emotional contagion, and more willingness and better aptitude for expressing feelings. Not only are women twice as likely as men to suffer psychological depression and anxiety, they are more apt to complain about their condition and to seek counseling. Women are less stoic than men. Being more sensitively and attentively responsive to their own feelings, women suffer more psychosomatic ills, are more hypochondriacal, more frequently visit physicians, and become sick more often. Women have a lower threshold of pain or tolerance of discomfort for both psychologic and physiological reasons (e.g., brain chemical production and physical endurance). Studies comparing the sexes have shown that women, while quite intimate with their emotional states, are less familiar with the capabilities, capacities, and working responses of their bodies (perhaps owing to fewer and less extreme physical challenges) and so are quicker to emotionally respond with greater suspicion to unusual or unpleasant physical changes. Psychologically speaking, women offer itemized and detailed descriptions of their psychological symptoms of depression, whereas men make more general statements about the quality of their lives and how things are not going as desired or expected. A 1989 Swedish study showed that male managers at a car manufacturing plant quickly unwound at home: their blood pressure dropped, and their noradrenalin levels subsided. This was not true of the female managers, whose nervous systems stayed agitated well into the evening. These and many other studies indicate that women do not cope with stress as well as men do.

## Aromatherapy for Women

The greater appeal that aromatherapy has for women correspondingly derives from the aforementioned psychological, biological, and behavioral factors. This is not only an aesthetic attraction to the cosmetic or beautifying aspects of aromatherapy but a genuinely therapeutic attraction as well. Women respond both to the aroma and to the therapy of aromatherapy, which unifies the sense of smell and emotional nature. Women are also more responsive to the hedonic and therapeutic features of various aromatherapy techniques (e.g., massage or cosmetology) and more amenable to the inhaled and transdermal psycho-physiological effects of essential oils. Owing to the uniqueness of female anatomy, physiology, and psychology, aromatherapy is an ideal holistic health system for women. Indeed, it would seem that nature designed it so—that women, essential oils, and aromatherapy are made for each other.

## Smell and Personality

Even though one person may be more skillful then another at identifying odors or better able to discern them, we are all rather inarticulate on the subject, restrained by the sparse vocabulary available to translate or communicate our subjective impressions of odors. Odors have no names. As human beings, we tend to describe odors by comparison, by analogy, or metaphorically. Usually you begin by saying an odor smells "good" or "bad," which of course merely means you like or dislike it. This reveals next to nothing about the substance's nature or its actual merits, effects, and properties but only how you feel about it. You may say an odor smells "clean" or "fresh" or inevitably that it smells like something else or the other. Even while thinking we share a common, albeit limited, lexicon for odors, we cannot be sure that we have agreed upon the same terminology. We may not agree even on the presence of an odor, or about what it is or whence it originates, let alone how we feel about it. The possible variables can make odor evaluation extremely complicated.

Your opinion of an odor may depend upon accompanying events or circumstances that distract or disturb you, lessening your attention to the odor or intensifying it, either pleasantly or unpleasantly. Depending on their strength or significance, those events or circumstances may become permanently or temporarily associated with that odor or even similar odors, after which your feelings for the entire experience may remain within your subconscious memory and response. "Responses to smells are like old habits," says Dr. Trygg Engen, professor at Brown University and author of *Odor Sensation and Memory,* and are learned in association with a moment and remain inextricably linked to the mood of that moment. This is one way mitigating social or environmental conditions—outside interventions in the smell process—can affect your evaluation of a scent. Physiological changes do likewise—more often temporarily. Because of the satiation bodily response, the same food aroma that stimulates your appetite and incites sensations and feelings of hunger before you eat becomes less appealing—perhaps aversive—after you've eaten. A woman's experience during pregnancy provides another example of physiological alteration of smell perception. We must also be aware of the determining factors of age, gender, health, and race in a person's smell perception.

Then, too, there are unique phenomena associated with sensory deprivations and disturbances other than those of smell. Evidently, sightless people are better able than normally sighted people to identify odors but are actually less perceptive or aware of odors. It seems that the supposed hyperosmia of the blind has more to do with their heightened response to odors—intensified by their visual deprivation—than with any increased smell sensitivity or acuity. It may well be that aphoristic "sensory compensation" owes more to intensified emotional experience than to any real increase in functional proficiency. Otherwise, the loss of one sense is not truly compensated for by the others; indeed, it diminishes them, since the human sensory experience depends greatly upon interaction and reciprocal enhancement of all five physical senses.

Fundamentally, three essential factors exist in smell perception: the odor, your nose, and you—i.e., your cognitive mind, psychological moods, and other aspects of your personality. It follows that after smell differences and scent preferences are identified and categorized according to demographics, race, gender, and age, certain behavioral traits eventually emerge that allow for further classifications according to personality types. Studies linking perfume preferences to personality profiles, mood tendencies, and personal lifestyle are being done and no doubt will continue. Standard psychology type classifications (e.g., introversion/extroversion) will be reexamined in the context of what they may tell us about people's smell preferences and differences. Fragrance Foundation–sponsored studies—intended to provide the industry profitable insights into consumer behavior, choices, and responses to fragrance products—show that people have enhanced self-image and social confidence when they believe they are wearing a fragrance that other people like. These studies also show that varying attitudes and motivations regarding scent use may be associated for marketing purposes into two types of people: (1) those who select fragrances for the sake of social appearance and who are therefore emotionally swayed by advertisements and marketing promotions that attach to the purchased perfume or cologne a certain glamourous image, with which these people identify and which they expect to acquire and convey by wearing it, and (2) those more intrinsically motivated, who select fragrances more on the basis of their own responses to the scent and who are presumably less concerned with image than with expressing a truer, more personally representative identity or persona. More findings reveal that people who regularly and extensively use scents consider themselves to be extraordinarily "sensitive," especially by all the more positive connotations of that word: more romantic, emotionally or psychically responsive, more loving, more caring, more sympathetic. Fragrance users also have a magnified hedonic response to scents. Given what we have heretofore learned in this chapter, none of these findings ought to be surprising.

Despite all the general indications of research and experimentation, the subjective nature of one's own smell and unique body odor represents the ultimate challenge to aromatherapists, osmologists, psychotherapists, and the rest, promising to keep their professional insights and techniques inexact but nonetheless worthwhile. Human variety and individuality should warn us that standardization of diagnosis and treatment in health or medical care must give way to individualized treatment, just as the individualized prescription was envisioned in aromatherapy by Marguerite Maury. Everything we now know about human nature should likewise caution us about mass aromatherapy via environmental fragrancing. We ought to be wary of any impersonal therapeutics involving aromatic substances, lest aromatherapy fall prey to the same mechanistic, "conveyer-belt medicine" mentality that Dr. Valnet rightly condemns in his book and which is already too prevalent in conventional medical practice.

# 4

# Aromatherapy Today and Tomorrow: Theory and Practice, Issues and Debates

Since the 1970s, Maralyn Teare, marriage and family counselor and a clinical instructor of psychiatry at the University of Southern California in Los Angeles, has used fragrance to reliably treat hundreds of phobia sufferers. Across town, Dr. Hyla Cass, assistant professor of psychiatry at the UCLA School of Medicine, agrees that the advantageous use of fragrance and smell in the psychological healing process ought to be included in the training of medical doctors and psychotherapists.

Elsewhere, through his "Invincible Athletics" program (designed to promote peak athletic performance using Transcendental Meditation and Ayurvedic practices), Massachusetts chiropractor John Douillard prescribes essential oils and other therapies for professional bodybuilders, runners, skiers, and cyclists as well as for triathletes such as Scott Molina and Colleen Cannon. Molina was one of the world's dominant triathletes during the 1980s; Cannon has been the U.S. women's best short-course triathlete and ranked among the top three female triathletes in the world. Like others on Douillard's program, Cannon claims that her daily training regimen with essential oils and aromatherapy has markedly improved her health and athletic performance. Douillard has trained some 200 U.S. medical doctors and chiropractors, affiliated with guru Maharishi Mahesh Yogi's Ayurveda

Health Centers, in the art of treating patients with aromatherapy and other natural therapies.

Created by French-born aromatherapist Daniele Ryman, After-Flight Regulator essential oil blends, designed to overcome the effects of jet lag, have been available at hotels and the duty-free shop in Heathrow Airport's International Terminal in London. Today, two international airlines, Air New Zealand and Virgin Atlantic Airways, are providing each of their first-class and business-class passengers an "after-flight regulator kit"—a package of two 5-ml bottles, one labeled "Awake," the other "Asleep," each containing an essential oil formula developed by Daniele Ryman, Ltd. Intended for bath or shower use upon arrival at one's destination, the formulas supposedly help attune the body to local time, by either stimulating or soothing the senses—a simple choice made evident by circumstances and the bottles' labels. The idea was adopted by the airlines after a test group of some 2,000 frequent flyers reported favorable results.

In Japan, "the era of perfume dynamics has arrived," according to Masakuni Kiuchi, an engineer for Shimizu, one of the three largest, if not the largest, of Japanese architectural, engineering, and construction firms. Quickly responding to Japanese research showing enhanced efficiency and reduced stress among workers exposed to scents, Shimizu is one of an increasing number of construction firms that over the past few years have developed a computerized environmental fragrancing system to deliver such scents into the workplace, both their own and those of other businesses. Moreover, since the late 1980s, Shimizu has been designing new offices and hospitals to include Shimizu's "Aroma Generation System," whereby liquid fragrances compressed into mist are pumped into working or living quarters through air-conditioning ducts and vents. Scented environments are not entirely new in Japan, which has a long tradition of various social rituals using incense, but these days even the Tokyo Stock Exchange has taken to fragrancing its inside air each afternoon with peppermint essence to invigorate and refresh employees.

It seems that in Japan not only are new and old buildings being scented, but some peculiar consumer goods are also being manufactured, among them an alarm clock that uses a built-in fan to blow a "forest scent" shortly before awakening the sleeper, a futon dryer that also spreads a floral fragrance over the bedding, and scent-infused pantyhose, all of which are now available for export to Europe and the United States. Is Japan merely giving us a whiff of our own medicine, or is this a sniff of things to come? In

Japan, Europe, and America, some people hope the latter is so. Others have real doubts and reservations, even fears, about this "era of perfume dynamics" in an increasingly fragrant society. More specifically, many think that the very idea of environmental fragrancing stinks.

## ENVIRONMENTAL FRAGRANCING

In early 1992, urged by the Citizen Commission on Human Rights (an arm of the Church of Scientology), a Massachusetts state legislator introduced a bill to ban any use of perfumes to "covertly control the behavior of others." The CCHR-sponsored ban would specifically prohibit the secret or subliminal use of aromas, scents, perfumes, or fragrances in businesses and public places. While citing the Japanese for already implementing such practices to increase worker productivity, the CCHR is also responding with alarm to current U.S. research aimed at developing scents to be vented into the New York City subway system to "induce a chemical euphoria as a method of reducing aggression." Is this a case of paranoia, or is environmental fragrancing an impending social problem requiring preemptive social or political action? Historical precedent for the CCHR's legitimate concern and for government intervention already exists, dating back to ancient Greece and Rome. Of course, some concerns about the effects of fragrances are less legitimate than others.

Some years ago, upon suffering a migraine headache she claims was caused by contact with a magazine scent sample, a New York woman, rather than sensibly avoiding such contact in the future (even assuming that the magazine was solely or partly responsible for her headache), petitioned her state legislator, who subsequently introduced a bill requiring scent samples in magazines sold in New York state to be sealed. More recently, according to *The Wall Street Journal*, employees at a "scent-free" New Jersey insurance agency have been prohibited from wearing fragrant cosmetics, including hair spray. "People are fed up with fragrances; they're so pervasive and intrusive," insists a New Jersey environmental health group activist who distributes buttons proclaiming "Perfume Pollutes." In apparent agreement, a San Francisco theatre chain has removed the air fresheners from all fourteen of its theatre restrooms. Meanwhile, in Marin County, California, the "National Foundation of the Chemically Hypersensitive," trumpeting its protection of the innocent from the evils of cologne and after-shave lotion, has demanded that designated "fragrance-free zones" be required in all restaurants and state-owned buildings. Julia Kendall is one of the more extreme activists in the group; because personal perfumes make her ill, she wants them prohibited everywhere. Based upon her own peculiar aversion to scents (the mere approach of someone wearing perfume causes her jaw to tighten, leaves her gasping for breath, and eventually gives her a severe headache), Kendall extrapolates that perfume is a public menace. The same sort of extended interpretation of personal experience characterizes the other members of her group. (Indeed, it is typical human behavior among various kinds of grievance groups.) Susan Molloy, who attends public meetings carrying an oxygen mask and tank, believes that scented personal products worn by others infringe upon her air space and that she is being unfairly driven from society by their presence. Terri White, executive director of the ironically named Center for Independent Living, and a backer of Molloy and her cause, desires that warning signs be posted on all buildings to deny entrance to anyone who wears perfume or whose clothing may be carrying the odor of smoke, dry cleaning, or fragrances. She wants the "chemically hypersensitive" to be legally represented as another disability or handicapped group and given protection under federal law.

These events in New York, New Jersey, and California, reported to illustrate a point, also require commentary. The elevation of a person's "victim status," which is established by one's membership in a specially designated social grievance group, has become a highly competitive and often highly profitable exercise in our increasingly contentious and litigious society. A tiny minority with an unfortunate idiosyncrasy and an overactive imagination, the "chemically hypersensitive" have literally raised that exercise to an art form by their hysterical claims of dangerous "second-hand scents" and unreasonable demands for odor bans and "fragrance-free zones" (as if such things were truly possible). The "chemically hypersensitive" (who, no doubt, are emotionally hypersensitive, since odor allergy is one of the more plainly psychogenic or psychosomatic ills) are now counted among those odd few factional groups who, rather than seeking individual solutions for their personal problems, instead demand that the larger society adapt, hinder, or inconvenience itself for their sake, regardless of the actual merits or consequences of their cause. Those advocating various forms of academic "right-thinking" or politically correct speech may soon be joined by "smell-patrol" zealots who intend to exploit hyperdysosmia by sniffing out offenders. It is instructive, however, that these phenomena and other idiosyncratic or otherwise incidental allergic reactions to scents and fragrances are neither attributable to aromatherapy nor the consequence of pure essential oils. Yet, while we recognize that synthetic scents or isolated, artificial ingredients are more likely to invite or provoke hypersensitivity or severe allergic response, such adverse reactions are hardly pandemic and form no basis for government restrictions upon personal odor or behavior. They certainly do not require the creation and advancement of yet another social cause, or public awareness campaign, or a new "victim class" of citizens. Nevertheless, what might happen if the same artificial, chemical scent ingredients were not randomly worn by individual people but instead were deliberately sprayed into public arenas is another matter altogether. Entirely new and truly public health risks would be created, some obvious and some not so obvious, which we will explore. But environmental fragrancing presents more than a social health problem; it creates an ethical predicament involving social and personal liberty that must be equally addressed.

## The Objectives of Environmental Fragrancing

The ostensibly benign objectives of "ambient fragrancing," as it is sometimes called, are essentially these: (1) to increase or enhance aesthetics, (2) to optimize performance and creativity at large, and (3) to improve air quality—that is, to relieve the multisymptomatic health problems of "sick building syndrome," so named because it is thought to be acquired by inhabiting tight, poorly ventilated homes and offices that inhibit the circulation of fresh air. The term now generally refers to health problems arising from occupying any stale, denatured or deenergized artificial or closed environment, especially those in which low-level toxic emissions (from rugs, paints, etc.) and unfiltered proliferating microorganisms are vented, usually through air conditioning systems. In actuality, according to latest statistics provided by a National Institute for Occupational Safety and Health study of 529 buildings, inadequate ventilation is the primary cause (53 percent) of poor indoor air quality. Inside or outside contaminants account for 15 percent and 10 percent, respectively. Microorganisms are responsible for only 5 percent of indoor air contamination; building materials cause only 4 percent. Unknown causes account for the remaining 13 percent.

As a new element of interior design (which already incorporates lighting, sound, color, and space), "sensory engineering"—as Sivon Reznikoff, professor at Arizona State University terms it—would design fragrancing to match or otherwise suit the needs of any architectural structure or interior environment. The expected results would include increased individual and social performance (memory, organization, mental acuity), job satisfaction, compliant cooperation, personal incentive, heightened vigilance, and accuracy. Immediately, one wonders how such a grandiose plan would account for a wide spectrum of individual needs, tolerances, and choices and about how it would require consensus of the targeted participants. Experimental scientific evidence or expert opinion about the "valuable results" of the plan might be initially convincing, but because human smell is a deeply subjective, personal, and diverse phenomenon, hardly uniform in preference and response, the plan is bound to elicit objections from the "fragrance-free" crowd, arouse suspicions of behavior modification and mind control, and meet resistance from just plain folks who have their familiar habits and own aesthetic ideas about how a particular environment ought to smell—and also their own ideas about what's good for them. Do people want artificial scents pumped into movie theatres to achieve the emotional effects desired by theatre owners and film makers? We've had "sensurround" and 3-D; what of "aroma films" that subliminally influence behavior or overtly enhance or obscure the expected odors of popcorn, candy, or the crowd itself? How potent must those "aroma film" scents be? Odors do not become consciously perceptible until quite strong, but they are always subconsciously effective—and just as effective even when undetectable by the nose.

## Scent Plans

A central problem with implementing any public plan or social strategy involving smell, whether intended to resolve health and aesthetic concerns or requirements, or designed to produce a particular performance result or behavioral response, is that everybody's sense of smell is different. Indeed, everyone is different in a variety of important ways. Because of that, proper scent selection, itself requiring wisely intelligent judgement, becomes more problematical. As Susan Knasko at Monell Chemical Senses Center observes, some people can smell only some of the ingredients in any given perfume, while others cannot smell any ingredients at all. Hence, the response to and effects of an odor, cognitively or subliminally, may be different. Knasko illustrates her point by saying that only half the population can smell androstenone, and among those who can, half perceive it as a subtly pleasant odor, while the rest say that it smells strongly disgusting. Maralyn Teare, citing her own experiential research, adds that all scents do not work on all people: "Scent is very person-specific; what may work for you may not work for someone else."

This uncertainty has not deterred environmental fragrancing in Japan where, beginning several years ago, Shimizu has devised at least twenty varieties of a "scent plan" to anticipate its clients' requests and better suit their business needs for greater efficiency or stress relief. For example, Shimizu says that a bank has specific needs requiring invigorating scents (e.g., lemon) in working areas to alert the staff, and calming scents (e.g., lavender) for bank customers. (If the novel idea that a bank can have "needs" is not curious enough, there also seems to be the implication that an alert bank staff needs some means to subdue its customers.) In partnership, Shimizu and Takasago, Japan's largest fragrance company, have implemented their scent plans for subliminal environmental fragrancing based upon the brain-wave research of Professor Shizuo Torii of the Toho University School of Medicine. Maybe the subliminal aspect of the scent plan is to tactically avert individual objections to the scents, but it has not escaped the attention of the Citizen Commission on Human Rights, which cites the Japanese in its campaign and support for legislation to prohibit the practice of subliminal fragrancing in Massachusetts.

In the earlier years of its joint venture development of Shimizu's Aroma Generation System and scent plan, Takasago conducted a series of experiments testing the efficiency of computer and word-processing operators. Takasago found, after thirteen operators were monitored eight hours a day for a month, that per-hour punching errors were reduced by nearly 21 percent when lavender scent was released into the office air, reduced by 33 percent using jasmine, and reduced by 54 percent using lemon scent. By reducing errors, the scents had increased work efficiency and productivity; increasing improvement was shown by the use of a more stimulating scent. One wonders, given the disparate results of lavender and lemon, how the apparent trade-off between lowering work stress (with lavender) at a cost of 33 percent reduced efficiency and productivity (as compared with lemon) is to be considered. Other questions arise: Would the effect of this ambient fragrancing diminish by habituation after continual exposure over a longer period of months? Other than habituation, what are the long-term health effects of continuous exposure to artificial scents? The questionable use of synthetic or denatured scents in environmental fragrancing is virtually guaranteed by the fragrance industry's large investment and involvement in the idea. (Takasago's "aromatherapy" fragrance creations for Japanese and American cosmetic companies, such as Avon, said to be based on aromatherapy principles, are not likely based entirely on essential oils.) Answering for the well-being of the participating keypunch operators, Junichi Yagi, a senior vice president of S. Technology, Shimizu's Massachusetts subsidiary, said that they enjoyed the fragrances, adding, "They reported feeling better than they did without it." Yagi also maintains that the fragrances were selected according to the principles of aromatherapy. The distinction here is that utilizing the principles of aromatherapy does not necessarily guarantee or require the use of the products of aromatherapy—pure essential oils—unless, of course, one believes, as do true aromatherapists, that the use of odorous substances other than genuine essential oils somehow violates those principles.

At the Kajima Corporation, another large Japanese construction company in Tokyo, another systemized "scent plan" adapted to the seasons, the weather, and the time of day cyclically emits scents to influence employees throughout each day. In the late 1980s, Kajima's scent plan was conceived by Shiseido, Japan's largest cosmetics manufacturer, and originally installed and tested in a then new three-building complex in Tokyo that holds a thousand Kajima employees. At first, oddly blending the separate principles of aromatherapy and democracy, Shiseido selected the fragrances to be used according to the scent preferences of the Kajima employees. For example, since jasmine was preferred more by women than by men, that fragrance would be used in offices where women constitute the majority, said Shiseido spokeswoman, Yukiko Fukuda.

The Kajima complex was centered on an atrium (plants and a waterfall) that can be seen from any one of the six lounges or the single meeting room nearby, into which a "forest scent" is pumped, thus enabling employees to breathe and view the "great outdoors" while still indoors. Otherwise, via the air conditioning unit, trees in the interior garden are made to emit a refreshing citrus aroma in the morning, a calming floral scent as the work day actually begins, and a supposedly invigorating (?) scent of cypress during lunch hour.

The Shiseido-Kajima partnership has sold dozens of environmental fragrancing units in Japan at $8,000 each. That seems inexpensive by comparison with Shimizu's customized systems, which cost about $20,000 per room, according to Junichi Yagi, whose Boston-based S. Technology subsidiary is preparing systems for sale in this country. Whether Shimizu's marketing strategy meets the same opposition elsewhere in the United States that it has encountered in Massachusetts remains to be seen. In Japan, meanwhile, people seem less concerned about being "led around by the nose" than they are about national corporate success and smart business. It is instructive to remember, however, that Japan is a small nation (slightly smaller than California) with a homogeneous population (99.4 percent Japanese) that, despite a century of Western modernization, has a long history of social and behavioral conformity and traditional acceptance of "social aromatics" in public rituals.

## Subliminal Shopping

"We've long controlled other parts of the retail environment, such as lighting, temperature, and decor," says J'Amy Owens, Seattle office president of Retail Planning Associates. "Now, we're finally realizing the influence smells can have on buying habits. Used properly, they can be a very powerful tool." As an environmental psychologist at Monell Chemical Senses Center, Susan Knasko has observed how scents make shoppers linger. Placing potpourri in a jewelry store during the 1990 Christmas holiday season made shoppers stay in the store longer, but they did not necessarily buy more jewelry. Yet, Knasko says, "Manipulating the ambiance through scent could be as powerful as setting a mood with lights or music." That is exactly how Mark Peltier, founder of Aromasys in Richfield, Minnesota, views environmental fragrancing. "This is olfactory Muzak," beams Peltier. "This is very, very big," which is how Peltier hopes his sales of "mood-altering fragrance systems" (ranging from $100 desktop models to $10,000 centralized units) will grow. His first commercial system has already been installed in the Miami Marriott Hotel, and he has received requests from several companies and universities, most frequently asking him to induce alertness, relaxation, and refreshment. Peltier reports that to "perk people up" he offers a blend of peppermint, lemon, eucalyptus, rosemary, and pine; to calm them down, he uses lavender and clove with "floral notes and a whiff of woodland"; and to refresh, he blends "citrus notes with pine and eucalyptus." (Without critically commenting upon Mr. Peltier's selective judgement, we needn't conclude that his "aromatherapy" is based solely upon essential oils.)

Dr. Alan R. Hirsch, director at the Smell and Taste Treatment & Research Foundation in Chicago, Illinois, is likewise "convinced smell is going to be the Muzak of the '90s, as more retailers realize how easily it can enhance their stores." For example, on the basis of his own study, Hirsch claims that shoppers in floral-scented shoe salesrooms are not only more apt to buy, but also more likely to pay more for athletic shoes than they otherwise would. Hirsch asked volunteers to give their opinion of one pair of Nike tennis shoes in a floral-scented room and another pair in a room with ordinary filtered air. Eighty-four percent of the participants preferred the pair in the floral-scented room; 10 percent were even willing to spend $10 more for the shoes. "Many of the subjects later said that they couldn't even tell that the floral scent was present, but they still liked the shoes in that room better," says Hirsch, adding "I'm definitely not endorsing the use of subliminal odors as a marketing tool, but it's clear that smells affect our perceptions and behavior, even if we can't smell them consciously."

In Britain, scientists at Warwick University are developing scents for a group called Marketing Aromatics, designed to influence staff and customers in work environments for everything from stress reduction to use of scented company stationery with a "corporate odor identity," all tailormade for each business's needs. So-called "signature scents" are becoming prevalent on both sides of the Atlantic. Victoria's Secret, a lingerie chain store and mail-order house, has adopted a potpourri scent for its feminine identity. Knot Shops tie stores emit a fragrance blend of spice, leather, and tobacco to convey masculinity. Dr. Hirsch's Smell and Taste Treatment & Research Foundation has been hired by one of the "Big Three" U.S. automobile manufacturers to develop a showroom scent that will increase car sales. Marketing Aromatics is doing the same while also secretly testing its mood-altering ideas in more than a hundred British stores, including department stores and travel agencies. Is this sly subliminal manipulation or simply clever marketing salesmanship? As observed, retailers already extensively employ music for shoppers; but is it the same thing when retailers and vendors insert subliminal odors into their products and stores to induce customers to buy? Is subliminal fragrancing more or less devious than using hidden, subliminal video or audio messages to urge buying and discourage shoplifting? Is it deception when a creditor laces payment bills with a faintly musky, chemical pheromone intended to intimidate customers into paying their bills more promptly? This has been tried in Australia by a mail-order cosmetics company whose scented final-notice bills sent to delinquent debtors were paid 17 percent more readily and rapidly than were bills sent on untreated paper. Meanwhile, in Las Vegas, Nevada, scents are being used to increase slot-machine and other gambling revenues by relaxing players and thus encouraging them to take more chances.

## A Brave New World

Dr. Charles Wysocki is an olfactory research scientist at Monell who notes the unique immediacy of smell's access to the limbic system and brain: "Smell is our most intimate, individualistic sense," he says. "It is primitive, uneducated, and therefore vulnerable." He warns that human emotions, with which smell is associated, can be readily exploited through the use of odors, scents, fragrances, and aromas. Dr. Trygg Engen of Brown University cautions that aromatic mood control could backfire: "Studies have shown that unidentified odors make people anxious. Other studies have shown that if a person feels he is being controlled, even by perfume, he is likely to find the aroma disagreeable."

Dr. Susan Schiffman of Duke University also has expressed reservations about environmental fragrancing. After more than twenty years of using fragrances such as chocolate and apricot to help alleviate depression and anxiety and to reduce aggression in her patients, she says she is disinclined to mass-market her findings: "The most powerful and effective aromatic suggestions remain highly personal and idiosyncratic." Yet, contradictorily, Schiffman's research is leading exploration of environmental fragrancing to reduce aggression in New York City subways. "We have to find ways to reduce aggression," says Schiffman. "We're looking at whether we can pump certain odors into a subway to make people less violent" and also into prisons "to reduce stress," which many, like the Church of Scientology and its Citizen Commission on Human Rights, interpret to mean the experimental mind control of a literally captive audience. Like so many others whose research is financially supported by the fragrance industry via its Fragrance Research Fund, Dr. Schiffman envisions many potential uses for fragrances, saying that scientific evidence gathered in sponsored studies by the FRF (for which Dr. Schiffman has served as scientific director) indicates a vast range of clinical, developmental, sociological, and physiological applications. Long before, in 1985, Henry Walter enthusiastically agreed, speaking as the chairman of the board of International Flavors & Fragrances in New York, the world's largest producer and supplier of scents. The IFF has made a multimillion-dollar commitment to research, investing huge sums of money in grants to universities, research centers, and individuals since the Fragrance Research Fund began in 1982. "We're putting our money where our nose is," remarked Walter, who likened the burgeoning market of fragrance products for "aromatherapy" to, in his own words, "the beginning of antibiotics." "We envision a zillion different possibilities," added Walter, including pumping stimulating aromas into schools to wake people up. But in this brave new world of odors envisioned by and divided between the synthetic fragrance industry and the conventional medical establishment, there is little or no room for traditional, holistic aromatherapy or real essential oils.

# PRETENDERS TO THE THRONE

## Aromatherapy vs. "Aroma-chology"

While riding the recent wave of interest in aromatherapy, the fragrance industry long ago adopted a strategy to distance itself from any recognition of essential oils, instead exploiting for its own purposes aromatherapy's growing popularity. A nonprofit organization formed in 1949 by the international perfume industry, today's New York–based Fragrance Foundation is still headed by top executives of such companies as Avon, Estée Lauder, Chanel, and Unilever and is membership supported by virtually every fragrance company (both manufacturers and suppliers) in the United States as well as by the associate membership of several big-name magazines (e.g., *Elle, Newsweek, Rolling Stone, Playboy,* and *Penthouse*). In 1982, the Foundation established its Fragrance Research Fund, a tax-exempt branch to promote scientific research into the effects of perfume upon human behavior. The FRF has funded numerous university, medical center, and individual studies (on sleep, performance, etc.) such as those by Peter Badia, Ehrlichman and Halpern, Dember and Warm, and the Memorial Sloan-Kettering Cancer Center. Significantly, for reasons that will soon become more obvious, the FRF does not include actual aromatherapists, and little or no research funding is expended toward investigating the therapeutic properties or value of essential oils.

The Fragrance Foundation prefers to explain the activity of perfumes (and that of essential oils) as a strictly psychological phenomenon rather

119

than physiological (or, more fashionably, "pharmacological") because the FF worries about possible drug classification of its products by the FDA requiring the fragrance and perfume industry to conduct more expensive regulatory testing. Furthermore, for financially motivated and commercially competitive reasons, the fragrance industry has no interest in substantiating the uniquely superior qualities and advantages of pure, natural essential oils and favorably contributing to the reputation and legitimacy of aromatherapy. Indeed, in disassociating itself from aromatherapy, the Fragrance Foundation, in 1988, coined a new term, "aroma-chology," to define its objectives. As explained by Annette Green, the FF's executive director, "aroma-chology" not only helps the Foundation distinguish itself from what Green refers to as the "New Age" incense and crystal-carrying crowd but cleverly maintains the link between fragrance and psychology while avoiding aromatherapy. "We stress the difference between what we do and aromatherapy," said Green in 1991. "Aroma-chology is basically a new science, and the response we've received from the academic community has been enthusiastic and international in scope. We've been funding various studies since 1982." The primary objective of the Foundation's huge ten-year research investment has been the development, large-scale manufacturing, and mass-marketing of aroma-chology products and what Green describes as "behavioral fragrances" for consumers, beginning with "stress-relief" formulas such as those now produced by Avon and Estée Lauder.

Aromatherapy and modern perfumery have long debated the comparative efficacy of natural and artificial aromatics. It remains aromatherapy's position that for genuine, healthful, long-term therapeutic results, only pure essential oils should be used. Modern perfumery maintains that there is no difference, that synthetic perfumes and isolated aromatic chemicals are the same as natural aromatic substances. Lately, perfumery's argument has been advancing in a crescendo of opinion. "It's lovely to say natural is better, but studies are showing that most people can discriminate only three components in a mixture," asserts Susan Schiffman, seemingly dismissing not only the more intelligent complexity of nature's products but also what has been otherwise discovered about essential oils, human olfaction, and the influence of subliminal odors. For Eugene P. Grisanti, speaking as chairman and president of International Flavors & Fragrances in 1990, public preference for natural substances is a public misperception. "It's the forest versus a petrochemical derivative," said Grisanti, "but both are chemicals.

There's nothing magical about it." There is, however, a new motivation in the fragrance industry's argument for artificial and isolated ingredients, although there is certainly nothing original in or about the "new science" of "aroma-chology." What is new is the Fragrance Foundation's admitted goal to have "aroma-chology" supplant aromatherapy in the public mind and market place. Previously, peaceful coexistence between aromatherapy and modern perfumery had been maintained by their serving different needs and ends. With the Foundation's declaration of intent for "aroma-chology," that is no longer the case.

## The Unholistic Alliance

For its "aroma-chological" raid on the aromatherapy market, the fragrance industry has enlisted the powerful medical establishment as its ally. Using a dual strategy of eradication and absorption, the scientific medical establishment (the American Medical Association, the pharmaceutical companies, et al.) has been waging its own decades-long war against what it refers to as "alternative therapies," such as homeopathy, chiropractic, acupuncture, herbology, and the health food industry, all of which are impediments to the medical establishment's agenda to monopolize America's health and medical care. For example, having failed to make the kind of merging inroads into chiropractic that it had made into osteopathy, the medical establishment shifted its strategy from absorption to eradication. On August 27, 1987, after an eleven-year court struggle to evade criminal charges of violating federal antitrust laws, the AMA was found guilty by a federal court of conspiring "to contain and eliminate the chiropractic profession." Also implicated as guilty co-conspirators were the American College of Surgeons and the American College of Radiology. The court found that as early as September 1963 the AMA sought the complete elimination of the chiropractic profession by arranging and spreading a professional, research, and educational boycott among other medical organizations and by deploying a paid staff of agents (lawyers, doctors, et al.) to publicly malign chiropractic with libelous, invidious name-calling. Even earlier, in October 1961, speaking on behalf of the AMA at a public meeting in Washington, D.C., a prominent AMA official openly solicited law-enforcement agencies, like the U.S. Department of Justice and the Federal Trade Commission, to assist the medical profession in "stemming the tide of such things as chiropractic" and help create an exclusive medical establishment. The apparent irony that the FTC was established to prevent just such professional business monopolies seems to have escaped the AMA representative.

Tactically, the medical establishment exercises its considerable political clout by advocating oppressive legislation to inhibit alternative therapies and by flexing its bureaucratic muscle—the FDA—to harass, threaten, or persecute the competition, which now includes aromatherapy. The fragrance industry and the medical establishment share a disdain for aromatherapy and a jealous desire to occupy or eradicate aromatherapy's market. But beyond that, they see an immediate opportunity to dominate newly created and highly profitable markets that capitalize on aromatherapy's appeal while excluding aromatherapy itself. The fragrance industry, for example, can see huge dollar signs in supplying the burgeoning commercial demand for environmental fragrancing with synthetic scents, just as is being done in Japan.

The unholistic alliance was formed in the laboratory. By sponsoring olfactory research with large financial grants to medical centers and university psychology departments, the fragrance industry gains scientific and academic credibility for its "aroma-chology" products and learns new ways to exploit smell by perfumery, environmental fragrancing, and other scented products. It may be thought, too, that by earning the gratitude of the scientific medical community, the fragrance industry is less likely to arouse the scrutiny of the FDA. Not only is "aroma-chology" legitimized by the industry's association with universities and individual psychologists and psychiatrists, many of whom serve the industry as consultants, but the psychologists and their departments gain steady, ample funding for their behavioral experiments involving olfaction, from which medical science learns ways to develop new "aroma-drugs" for human behavior modification. Not content with the prospects of modifying individual psychological behavior or collective group behavior through mood-altering environmental fragrancing pumped into subways, schools, and prisons, medical science also conceives new medical procedures to chemically or surgically alter olfaction itself. Dr. Schiffman is among those who recognize the mutual advantages of the FRF's large financial investment toward olfactory research, which she hopes will someday make it possible for medical science to surgically implant specific odor receptors into the olfactory membranes of humans to achieve a desired olfactory response. Increased receptor implants may be used to reverse smell atrophy or anosmia in the aged and treat other smell disorders as well. Knowledge of olfactory receptor shapes will improve scientists' ability to synthesize certain fragrances having specific behavioral effects, and that knowledge can be used to assist the perfume and pharmaceutical manufacturing of "behavioral fragrances" and "aroma-drugs."

## If You Can't Beat `Em, Eat `Em: The Strategy of Eradication and Absorption

Yet, the scientific medical establishment continues to publicly dismiss aromatherapy as a nonsensical health fad or, at best, an experimental treatment, disregarding man's universal 5,000-year experience with aromatics and despite the many past and current studies and observations. "Maybe in the future, it could turn out that some of these medical claims [for aromatherapy] are true," said University of Cincinnati professor of anatomy and cell biology Robert Gesteland in May 1991, "but at this point there aren't any good experiments to support them." The 1991 edition of the AMA's Encyclopedia of Medicine gives the following description of aromatherapy:

> Recently, interest in aroma therapy has been rekindled along with other alternative therapies. . . . Practitioners claim that the treatment can be used for a range of disorders, but that it is particularly effective in psychosomatic and stress-related disorders. . . . There is no conclusive scientific evidence that the benefits achieved are greater than those achieved by the power of suggestion.

But then, the conventional allopathic medical profession says much the same thing about other alternative therapies, regardless of the facts or evidence. The medical establishment's opinions might be more convincing if it first applied the same "scientific evidence" standard to the multitude of over-the-counter and prescription drugs and high-tech medical procedures that, while wildly profitable, have yet to be shown of clinical value or efficacy. Meanwhile, numerous independent studies and evaluations, some by our own government, have shown many drugs and procedures to be ineffectual or of dubious worth, if not otherwise risky or counterproductive. For example, a study reported in 1991 by the *Journal of the American Medical Association*, found that children administered Amoxacillin for middle-ear infections had recurrence rates 2 to 6 times higher than children who were not given the antibiotic. At one point, the Office of Technology Assessment estimated that "only 10 to 20 percent of all procedures currently used in medical practice have been shown to be efficacious by controlled trial." Whereas most holistic or naturopathic techniques and remedies have been successfully used for hundreds—even thousands—of years, most medical drugs and surgical procedures are quite recent, and many are just a few years old. Yet, the medical establishment would have us believe that naturopathy, Ayurveda, herbology, aromatics, acupuncture, and the rest, which together have satisfied at least 90 percent of the world's health care needs, are unproven alternative therapies that are counter to the laws of science and nature. In applying a double standard of scientific evidence to alternative therapies, the conventional medical establishment gives new meaning to the term "double-blind study" by exhibiting an unscientific prejudice and a profound ignorance concerning the alternative therapies it extemporaneously condemns. Most orthodox medical physicians learn or are taught virtually nothing about alternative therapies, even those like herbology and nutritional therapy that are nearest to conventional medicine. Separate surveys of 127 medical schools reveal that only 25 to 46 offer educational courses in nutrition, let alone instruction in acupuncture, aromatherapy, or any of the other naturopathic systems of healing. Consequently, allopathic or medical physicians and personnel are typically unqualified and unprepared to evaluate or utilize alternative therapies. They see no profit or professional advantage in learning or recommending them, and they are given no incentive to do so by the medical establishment—quite the reverse: they are frequently dissuaded and discouraged from doing so. Dissenters, or those who for independent reasons educate themselves or otherwise fairly investigate alternative therapies, are subject to censure, and if they persist so far as to espouse or adoptively practice such heretical therapies, they risk persecution or excommunication by the medical establishment.

The scientific medical establishment's reaction to the perceived threat of a competitive alternative therapy follows a "3-R" tactical policy: (1) repudiation—deny its very existence, if possible; otherwise, deny its validity or importance; (2) ridicule—deride and belittle it as worthless, possibly dangerous "quackery"; (3) resistance—attempt eradication by regulatory legislation and strong-arm tactics aimed directly against practitioners, providers, suppliers, and consumers. Implementation of this tactical policy must always appear to be "in the best interests of the public" (i.e., to protect the public's health, safety, and welfare) and not seem to be a self-serving campaign to protect the monopolistic professional and business interests of the conventional medical community.

The absorption half of the strategy operates when the scientific medical establishment acknowledges, but never publicly admits, the actual therapeutic value and merits of the alternative therapy. If an alternative therapy is estimated to be profitable to some segment of the conventional medical community, the medical establishment will confiscate, adapt, rename, and repackage that therapy and its products for marketing to the public—but under the "safe, qualified, and professional" administrative control of medical science and its adherents. This brings us back to aromatherapy and "aroma-chology."

While the fragrance industry and medical establishment together recognize olfaction's importance and the power of odorants to influence human behavior, they must, for their own professional advantage and financial incentives, continue to disavow aromatherapy and essential oils. Essential oils are regarded as unnecessarily expensive for the purposes of the fragrance industry, which can accomplish its commercial objectives more predictably and cost-effectively by using inferior but less expensive synthetics. Medical science likewise dismisses aromatherapy for competitive reasons and because essential oils are unpatentable, widely and unrestrictedly available natural substances that present far less profit potential than can be realized through medical science's exclusive pharmaceutical patenting, production, and distribution of synthetics and artificial "odor drugs."

Only a thin layer of constitutional and legislative protection shields essential oils, vitamin and mineral supplements, herbs, and other nutritional and therapeutic natural substances from being completely restricted or reclassified as "drugs" by the FDA. The medical establishment is aggressively and assiduously attempting to destroy that layer of protection for reasons that are as plain as the nose on your face. Having the FDA ban or otherwise place the tools and products of natural, holistic therapies under the exclusive control of the conventional medical community would first drive those alternative therapies out of business. Next, those natural products that didn't disappear altogether from the market place would be more restrictively dispensed by the medical community, either on drugstore shelves or by prescription only. The more restricted dispensation would create higher profits not only from the sale of the confiscated substances but from both the old and "new" (merged or absorbed) therapies involving those substances.

## Over There

The climate for aromatherapy is thought to be less hostile and more prosperous in Europe than it is here in America. But even overseas, the same opposing forces are militating against aromatherapy and the use of essential oils. It should be understood that the dispute or antagonism between medical science (behavioral psychologists, chemists, allopaths) and naturopathic practitioners of aromatherapy does not simply derive from intellectual disagreements about methodology involving debabte over the relative merits of the analytical experimental approach and the experiential approach of holistic therapy. It arises from long-standing, profound ideological differences about healing and medicine and from professional bias and jealous rivalry over profit and power. It includes a broader debate over who will control social or national health and medical care and, in this particular case, who will seize control of the "new science" of "aromachology," "psycho-aromatherapy," "osmotherapy," or whatever one chooses to call it. In this debate, the incumbent medical establishment views aromatherapy as an upstart adversary.

Phytoaromatherapy continues to thrive and retain its appeal and popularity in Europe despite occasional setbacks. In France, phytoaromatherapy patients were once entitled to a tax reimbursement of 80 to 100 percent for all herbal and essential oil pharmaceutical preparations obtained through France's National Health Insurance. In 1990, the French government abruptly rescinded the cost refund, outraging the public and nearly ruining the entire phytoaromatherapy business, from practitioners on down to essential oil distributors and suppliers. Patients were forced to pay the full cost of prescriptions, initially causing a sharp drop in the demand for production and sale of essential oils. This adversely affected the growers of aromatic plants, laboratories, pharmacists, and phytoaromatherapists. Some companies went bankrupt, and many doctors experienced a drastic reduction in clientele. Phytoaromatherapy's recovery from this near disaster has been slow but steady, owing to the increasing public demand for natural remedies. By the time of this writing, the immense public and professional pressure on French officials to correct the outrage may have already led to government reinstatement of the tax refund. Meanwhile, since 1993, owing to increased interest in the efficacy of herbal drugs, or phytopharmaceuticals, German medical students have been required to study herbal medicine, which will include examination testing on phytotherapy.

In 1987, when it was reported that British prime minister Margaret Thatcher availed herself of aromatherapy treatments devised by Daniele Ryman and that other members of both parliamentary houses had also been frequenting Ryman's London clinic, it may have seemed that aromatherapy had truly arrived in Great Britain. Yet, despite these and other signs of the amazing progress and popularity of aromatherapy in England, and the remarkable success of British aromatherapists, the chasm between members of the British medical establishment on one side and the holistic practitioners and adherents of aromatherapy on the other remains deep and wide. The Olfaction Research Group at the University of Warwick in Coventry, England (where corporate-identity "signature scents" are being developed), is making attempts to span the gap of understanding between the two sides by using the group's own research and by arranging conferences at which all parties might share their findings and exchange viewpoints. The first International Conference on the Psychology of Perfume was held in 1986, followed by a second conference in July, 1991, organized by two university members of the group: Steve Van Toller, a psychologist, and George Dodd, a biochemist converted to aromatherapy, who is personally engaged in a struggle with the Medicines Control Agency (Britain's FDA counterpart) over licensing of natural "osmotherapy" products. (Van Toller and Dodd are co-editors of the book *Perfumery: The Psychology and Biology of Fragrance.*) Regrettably, indications from the conference and elsewhere are that there has been little or no improvement in the opinions and attitudes of those in the conventional scientific medical community toward aromatherapy. By the medical community's responses, ranging from amused condescension to incredulous hostility, it seems the best that can be presently hoped for is a grudging admission that alternative therapies, such as aromatherapy, have some redeeming value as "complementary" medicine. This was the conclusive evaluation of aromatherapy given by establishment physicians who, in the summer of 1985, attended the Alternative Medicine Exhibition in London. Among their observations was the recognition that alternative modalities have emerged from the public's grave dissatisfaction with both the mechanistic philosophy and the actual health care and service provided by the conventional medical profession. (As the successes and popularity of alternative therapies continue to mount and soar, so too does the volume of public complaints about modern medicine: practitioners who are arrogantly narrow-minded, insensitive, and uncommunicative; tests and procedures that are painfully repetitious, tedious, needlessly complicated, and outrageously expensive; treatments and medicines that are sickening, sometimes dangerously debilitating, and often aggravating and ineffective; and so on.) Included in its comments about alternative therapies, the physicians' report said, "Aroma therapy explores the olfactory sense by the use of essential oils which are not simply sniffed, but massaged into the entire body, an experience which must be singularly refreshing." The physicians conceded that one of aromatherapy's strengths is the rapport created between client and healer: "Such trusting and physical relationships can—as anyone who has derived benefit from massage knows—be infinitely soothing and rather different from some experiences at the hands of doctors. Lying down plus physical manipulation affords a unique opportunity to relax, concentrate, receive 'tender loving care,' talk through worries, and learn." Faint praise indeed.

## Second Opinions

As we've learned, not everyone in the medical science establishment or at the olfactory research centers scoffs at aromatherapy. Monell's Susan Knasko retains her skepticism of aromatherapy, attributing responses to suggestive expectation, but Dr. Gary Beauchamp, Monell's taste researcher, believes that essential oils are pharmacologically (physiologically) active, given that essential oils are lipid soluble and therefore capable of penetrating the skin and blood-brain barrier. Beauchamp conjectures that odorants may also travel up the olfactory nerves from the cilia on the nasal epithelium, in which case odor materials get closer to the central nervous system than just the lining of the nose.

At International Flavors and Fragrances in Union Beach, New Jersey, which conducts computerized analysis of natural odor components to create synthetics for perfume and fragrance products, Dr. Stephen Warrenburg, a psychophysiologist, works on "fragrance psychology," mostly to determine dichotomous like/dislike reactions to scents. There, Dr. Craig Warren and others at IFF have acquired what they regard as solid objective (machine-monitored) and subjective (self-reported or observed) evidence that their essential oil mixtures, administered topically (transdermally) or by inhalation, reduce anxiety and other stress-level emotions.

Meanwhile, psychology professor Howard Ehrlichman of the City University in New York has expressed some important doubts about the entire odor-olfaction process: "I certainly don't believe in anything as uncomplicated as presenting an odor to produce an automatic response," said Ehrlichman in 1985. "Think how complicated food is. When you're hungry, a garlic smell may make your mouth water; but if you're full, it may produce other feelings. . . . There are very, very few [odor] stimuli that have an immediate effect good or bad." If so, one wonders why his and other FRF-financed studies on olfaction and odors continue.

Dr. Gary Schwartz, professor of psychology and psychiatry at the University of Arizona in Tucson, replies, "I was a disbeliever—I thought it was unlikely that a specific fragrance could have a demonstrably relaxing effect in the laboratory. But it makes sense to me now." Schwartz says that while at Yale University he produced just such an effect with an "apple spice" scent. Yet another IFF grant recipient, Dr. Schwartz conducted his financed experiments over a five-year period at Yale, testing more than 400 subjects, before publishing the results in 1989. He noted that spiced apple had relaxing effects as measured in brain waves—in one subject's case, within a minute. In a separate study, spiced apple had a noticeable reduction effect on the stress levels of monitored subjects who were asked a series of questions intended to cause tension. The respiration, blood pressure, heart rate, and muscle tension of those exposed to the scent measured lower than in test subjects who received bursts of plain air.

Since arriving at the University of Arizona, Schwartz has turned his attention to studying subliminal scent, particularly the effects of "sick buildings" wherein, as Schwartz describes it, we are made to breathe a veritable soup of artificial chemicals. "The idea is that the nose can detect those molecules and that information is fed to the brain and does activate brain centers to make us feel queasy or uncomfortable." Schwartz adds that we would be unable to attribute our responses to any of these odors because of their subliminal existence. The idea of therapeutic odors is supported by Schwartz, yet predictably he never mentions or utilizes essential oils, referring instead to the synthetic scents provided by the modern organic chemistry labs of medical science and the fragrance industry. This last point is significant, because not only in the lab but in real life, synthetic odors are not simply intruding upon natural odors but are threatening to supplant them.

## Artificial Inhalation

Dr. Alan Hirsch of the Smell and Taste Treatment & Research Foundation has already concluded that our frame of reference for aromas is gradually drifting away from nature and toward manufactured compounds. Numerous clinical and observational studies can be recounted that indicate how the human nose is being deceived by manufactured odors, which, coupled with our modern urbanized detachment from nature, is causing confused and distorted identity associations between odors, tastes, and their sources. Dr. James A. Steinke, director of flavor development and application at Fries & Fries, a Cincinnati laboratory that compounds flavors for the food industry, notes: "People raised on strawberry Kool-Aid will prefer the Kool-Aid-type berry flavor over a completely natural berry. Actually, if you squished fresh berries and blindfolded these tasters, they would say it wasn't fruit."

That for a rapidly increasing number of human beings, an artificial "fruit flavor" represents what they now believe is the "real" scent and flavor of fruit, and that real fruit no longer smells "real," tells us something important about what Monell's Dr. Wysocki calls the "primitive, uneducated, and therefore vulnerable" nature of smell and about how the human nose and tongue, inundated with bogus odors and phony flavors, can be falsely satisfied by artificial stimuli that while "pushing the right buttons" and saturating the senses offer no therapeutic or nutritional benefits whatever. Artificial substances do this not by mere equal substitution for the real thing but by false exaggeration, which provides us more of the hedonic stimulus and response we like, even while providing us less of everything else we really need or expect. Often, only because they smell and taste like those things that are good for us, we are duped into eating, drinking, and smelling things that are not good for us.

As if ersatz scents masquerading as the real thing weren't enough of a problem, the cross-proliferation of scented products, "natural" or otherwise, further complicates our ability to correctly identify odors. "It's getting confusing," says Susan Knasko of Monell. "Everything is scented. Many people learn scents out of context and it's starting to affect my research." For some people, lemon scent means lemonade; for others it's furniture polish, and so on. Knasko reports that in research studies when subjects 18 to 45 years old smell pine scent, they often think it's a cleaning product or otherwise misidentify the odor as lemon because lemon and pine are so commonly mixed in cleaning and household products. The age range of her subjects is telling, since other studies reveal that younger generations are gradually being conditioned and acclimated to synthetic chemical odors which are rapidly replacing natural scents, fragrances, and aromas in our work and home, indoor and outdoor environments, food and beverages, toys, clothing, and other products. While contemplating the countless substances and materials of modern industrialism and technology that have been introduced to our olfaction during the latter half of the twentieth century, one begins to realize how present and future generations will be increasingly influenced emotionally, hedonically, and nostalgically by fabricated fragrances rather than by natural odors. What this portends is unknown, but the implications and consequences could be tremendous. Perfumers and flavorists are well aware of this olfactory shift observed by Dr. Hirsch and others. Having 10,000 mostly synthetic aromatic substances available to fashion fragrances, and 5,000 mostly artificial ingredients to fabricate flavors for packaged foods, the fragrance and food industries are quite busy furthering that trend.

## On the Wrong Scent

In producing their psycho-physiological effects, essential oils traverse the blood-brain barrier not only by virtue of their lipid solubility when utilized transdermally or by ingestion but also by triggering nerve impulses olfactorally when they are inhaled. This is not exclusive entry; other substances can do likewise. But since all odors are not created equal, the question is, what message, what information, does each offer or carry to the brain? Varied scientific processes of manipulating or tampering with naturally occurring matter or substances (whether genetically, chemically, molecularly, or atomically) can produce mutations, denatured or unnatural substances that are synthesized, isolated chemical constituents or artificial replications. Always there is the risk of imbalancing or somehow distorting the effects or character of the original that is being processed or imitated, consequently creating something that is less healthful, therapeutically effective, or valuable yet more psycho-physiologically active or potent in a narrow, limited, and disturbing way. This is often what likewise creates abnormalities of human response to such unnatural substances, ranging from simple allergies to toxicity or addiction. Considering what we've learned about olfaction, is it possible to become chemically and psychologically addicted to false scents? That is, can we learn to prefer or rely upon them more than we do natural aromas and fragrances? Judging by the human experience with numerous modern synthetic drugs variably classified as hypnotics, sedatives, tranquilizers, narcotics, stimulants, depressants, and hallucinogens, we ought to conclude that the answer is yes. First, to be effective, an inhaled "aroma drug" need only find the right receptor by imitating a natural substance. A potent enough synthetic odor would then operate in much the same way as oral, injected, and nasal drugs already do, by exaggerating hedonic response, intensifying the psycho-physiological stimuli and effects, and creating an increased desire for and eventual dependence upon the synthetic odor.

Some years ago, Professor Susan Schiffman of Duke University noted that a group of recently isolated olfactory receptors are the same receptors that bind Valium and Librium. (Chemically named diazepam and chlordiazepoxide, respectively, Valium and Librium are the two most frequently and profitably prescribed benzodiazapine tranquilizer-sedatives in the United States, where they are manufactured by the same pharmaceutical company.) "Now, they did not evolve over millions of years so they could be around to bind Valium when it was invented," says Schiffman, "so why are they there in our noses? My guess is that they might be there to bind things that we smell, natural substances that have a similar effect." A good guess, since human beings and other animal species have been using medicinal plants for countless thousands—indeed millions—of years.

## Nature's Pharmacy

> *The Most High hath created medicines out of the earth,*
> *and a wise man will not abhor them."*
> **Ecclesiasticus 38:4**

The native African people of Tanzania have traditionally used the *Vernonia amygdalina* bush to cure and prevent intestinal parasites and other gastrointestinal disorders. In 1987, primatologists discovered that Tanzania's chimpanzee population used the same bush for the same purposes. Since that year, researchers have indentified some fifteen plant species included in what they now refer to as "the pharmacopoeia of the apes," which is utilized not only by chimps but by howling monkeys, rhesus monkeys, and very likely all other ape species as well. These and other animal species have long ago discovered, in nature's medicine cabinet, therapeutic remedies, cures, and preventive medicines for whatever ails them. Scientists are now devoting special attention to zoopharmacognosy—the use of medicinal plants by animals—under the premise that what works for other primates, and mammals, may work for humans too. Chimps sometimes take early morning walks for as long as twenty minutes just to ingest the leaves of *Aspilia*, a member of the sunflower family, which scientists know is high in a red oil—thiarubrine-A—that destroys parasites, fungi, and viruses. Instinctively, the chimps know that too. After lab testing, biochemists are now discovering that thiarubrine-A kills cancer cells in the kind of solid tumors that most commonly occur in the breasts and lungs.

Like all survival skills, animal recognition of medicinal plants is an acquired ability combining inborn instinctive knowledge, sensory perception, imitation, and some trial and error—all part of the evolutionary natural selection process to maintain and improve the species. Howling monkeys in Costa Rica, like other animal species, smell and taste plants to distinguish the plants' qualities, and evaluate their medicinal worth as well as their potential dangers. Adult monkeys also instruct their young by searching for and administering certain medicinal plant leaves and roots. As a prophylactic measure, Tanzania's chimps eat more *Aspilia* and *Vernonia* during the rainy season than during other times. There is sufficient evidence to suggest that animals use plants for obstetric purposes, too. In humans and other primates, sperm carrying the female X chromosome last longer in an acidic medium, whereas sperm carrying the male Y chromosome outlive X-carrying sperm in an alkaline medium. To correctly regulate the species, primates like the howling monkey will instinctively ingest plant foods and substances just before and after mating that they do not otherwise eat, thereby becoming able to alter the pH conditions under which fertilization takes place. It seems that the plants' acid or alkaline compounds change uterine conditions, thereby affecting fetal gender. Too, other plants contain chemical compounds that influence female production of estrogen, which in turn affects estrus, or ovulation. This is quite like the knowledge acquired by humans, just as Dr. Valnet reminds us in his book: vervain, a flowering plant of the genus *Verbena*, family Verbenaceae, had been used in midwifery as an infusion to strengthen the uterus and ease labor, long before science discovered that vervain contains the compound verberin, a powerful uterine contracting agent.

It seems that early and primitive humans learned much from the animals about medicinal plants. According to ancient Navajo legend, the bear taught the tribe to use osha (*Ligusticum porteri*), which has a host of healing powers (including antimicrobial, antitoxin, stomachic, carminative, vermifuge, sudorific, and expectorant properties) for treating gastrointestinal ills, bacterial and viral infections, and other diseases. The Navajo and other native North American Indians also burn the plant as incense to ward off pathogenic and miasmic influences. (This practice is called "smudging" and the incense burner a "smudge pot.") Also known as "bear medicine" or "Indian parsley," osha is still used by tribes today, as it is by the bear. Alaska's great Kodiak bears will sometimes unearth and swallow osha roots, at other times chewing them open or into a mush to rub the plant's juices on their fur. Brown bears do likewise. It is now known that among its numerous chemical substances, *Ligusticum porteri* contains natural fungicides that also repel ticks and other parasites.

By the late nineteenth century, quinine, a bitter alkaloid extracted from the bark of the cinchona tree imported from South America to Europe, was routinely used to treat malaria and other febrile illnesses. In ancient Peru, the Indians had learned the medicinal benefits of eating cinchona bark by watching the puma. On the other side of the globe, in the Dutch East Indian ports of what is now Indonesia, malaria, which was rampant, was commonly treated with cinchona tree bark, as were other fevers and various nonfebrile ailments. There, a Dutch sea captain, by self-experimentation, found cinchona to be effective for his episodes of rapid and irregular heartbeat. His personal experience, described in 1914 medical literature by his European doctor, led to the isolation of quinidine, quinine's stereoisomer (molecular mirror image), which since has been used as a heart medication. Inevitably, chemists synthesized variants of the quinine molecule, creating quinine derivatives called antimalarial drugs (quinacrine, chloroquine, hydroxychloroquine) which soon replaced the natural constituent quinine in modern medical practice.

## In Search of Ecstasy

Animal behavior has also led man to the discovery of analgesics, sedatives, and stimulants. According to Ethiopian folklore, it was sometime in the tenth century that herdsmen first observed their goats leaping excitedly into the air after eating coffee beans. In Australia, eucalyptus was seen to quiet koala bears, which dine exclusively on the leaves of the tree, providing some indication of the mildly anesthetic, sedative properties of certain eucalyptus varieties, such as *Eucalyptus citriodora.*

In the search for natural healing agents, still more plants that provide pain relief or increase physical stamina and performance have been discovered, as well as plants having psychoactive capabilities to relieve anxiety and depression or to produce or enhance psycho-physiological states. Just as wild animals, to varying degrees, will venture outside their normal feeding range or alter eating habits to acquire and ingest such plants, modern man—the most complex biological organism on earth—has geographically and gastronomically widened the human range beyond that of other animals, coincidental with man's global exploration, travel and trade, and development of an extraordinarily omniverous diet. Nonetheless, Ronald Siegel, a pharmacologist whose specialty is psychopharmacology (the study of drug effects upon behavior) has concluded, after twenty years of observing dozens of animal species and human societies, that the drive to pursue intoxication is a common biological behavior throughout the animal kingdom, more particularly among mammals because of how the mammalian brain is wired, and especially among primates.

In his book *Intoxication: Life in Pursuit of Artificial Paradise,* Siegel asserts that although the drive to alter consciousness is an acquired motivation, it can be as powerful as innate, instinctive drives involving hunger, thirst, and sex. He relates that in the Canadian Rocky Mountains, bighorn sheep often climb the sheerest rock ledges just to sample the narcotic-like properties of the lichen growing there. African elephants seek out the fermented fruit of the native *Borassus* tree, from which they sometimes get staggering drunk. Further examples abound in nature. A potentially dangerous but highly potent medicinal herb of the nightshade variety, henbane (so called because it is readily fatal to chickens) has poisonous narcotic properties similar to those of belladonna, owing to certain alkaloid compounds. Yet, henbane is judiciously nibbled by other mammals that are more carefully aware of its numbing effects. Jimson weed, or "locoweed," which contains alkaloids found in henbane and belladonna (scopalamine, hyoscyamine, atropine), is an equally hazardous hallucinogen consumed by cattle and horses of the North American West, often with deadly results. Hallucinogenic mushrooms are favored by many wild species around the globe, just as catnip is favored by domestic felines around the house.

But we must carefully distinguish animal behavior from human behavior when it comes to the common pursuit of tranquilizers, narcotics, and other psychoactive substances. Although animals may sometimes suffer dire consequences, they have legitimate health purposes in seeking the effects produced by such dangerous plants. (In gauging the risks, wild animals seem to exercise greater restraint and better judgement than do more domesticated animals such as horses, chickens, or cattle.) Man's use of hallucinogenic mushrooms, peyote, marijuana, or opium often has entirely different motives. Animals are not idle or compulsive thrill-seekers hoping to "get stoned" or "get high" or to escape reality; neither do they have mystical or religious motivations to seek states of altered consciousness or spiritual ecstasy. The comparison is similar to the practical survival purposes for which animals use smell and scent, in contradistinction to the romantic, hedonically exotic or aesthetic motivations that often guide human olfaction. The differences become more dramatically clear when one considers how, unlike animals, humans are now capable of manufacturing their own synthetic drugs and then using them imprudently—which brings us to the core of a modern problem.

From one generation to the next, the Andean Indians of South America have regularly chewed coca leaves to stimulate and fortify themselves during long journeys and strenuous tasks. Coca is the same plant from which cocaine is synthesized. Yet, among the Andeans there are no documented cases of deaths occurring from overdose or abuse of this substance, no evidence of social decay or health problems. Meanwhile, modern civilized societies are plagued by heavy or habitual drug users who by snorting cocaine or smoking "crack" (or abusing other drugs) destroy themselves, their family or social relationships, and other members of society, and who commit crimes or otherwise burden society with their cocaine-addicted babies. One explanation may be the genetic differences between different peoples using a same or similar substance. For example, among racial and ethnic groups there are greater and lesser tolerances to alcohol and hence, varied probabilities of health risks, intoxication, or addiction that are largely predetermined genetically. Too, there are immense comparative differences in psychological stress between modernized, urban society and primitive or rural societies. Yet another major factor is the often foolish, disrespectful ways in which modern man handles natural substances. Explains Siegel:

What went wrong is that being the technologically sophisticated primates that we think we are, we've ripped apart these leaves, taken the chemicals out, concentrated them down, injected them into our bloodstreams, and then asked why we have a problem. We're taking some safe medicines, safe drugs, some relatively benign intoxicants, and we're turning them into poisons by changing the dosages and patterns of use.

Whether the discussion is about whole, natural foods versus processed foods containing additives, preservatives, and artificial flavors, or natural plant medicines versus synthetic drugs, it becomes clear that modern man has been led astray by the same wrong idea. In the similar debate over pure essential oils versus synthetic or isolated aromatic substances, we first should reject any attempt to ascribe pharmacological effects to essential oils as being a complete misapprehension of their nature and of the actual pharmacological effects of existing drugs or new "aroma drugs" proposed in the future.

Dr. Schiffman's guess is correct. Brain and olfactory receptors did not evolve over millions of years just to be there when Valium, Librium, or any other drug was invented. Drugs are imposters. Such drugs as tranquilizers and barbituates not only deplete or inhibit essential nutrients and cellular oxygen, they lead to addiction by the habituated tolerance or adaptation of the host organism—a more serious matter than tolerance of the microbe, as occurs with the use of antibiotics. Hence, psychoactive drugs require larger and more perpetual dosages until they become worse than imposters—they become usurpers. The costs and side-effects of such "therapy" can become enormous. They are usually paid for by mental, spiritual, and creative decline; nervous and behavioral disorders; loss of appetite, libido, or social awareness; and diminishment of sensory responses—all resulting from physical, psychological, and spiritual toxication.

It is instructive that the Citizen Commission on Human Rights's opposition to the notion of pumping "behavioral fragrances" into our prisons, schools, and subways is a continuance of the Church of Scientology's war against psychiatry or, more specifically, against what Scientology views as the psychiatric profession's misuse of mind-altering, psychoactive drugs that reduce people into zombies. It may first be recognized in this dispute that synthetic scents and artificial fragrances are another generation of imposters, which, if handled as drugs are and have been handled, could harm individuals and threaten society in much the same way. Do we need or want another generation of synthetic drugs—this time "behavioral fragrances" or "olfaction drugs"—that treat symptoms rather than people and will likely generate more personal and social problems than they resolve? It is incumbent on phytoaromatherapists to encourage the use and supply of natural botanicals and aromatics, to counter the disturbing modern trend toward synthetic scents and artificial substances, and to educate all concerned about the increasingly important need for authentic fragrances that have true therapeutic and aesthetic value.

## Aromatherapy Questions and Answers

In all capacities, essential oils, herbs, and other plant remedies provide a safe, sane, and healthful alternative to the synthetic products of the chemistry lab. Essential oils are foremost among those medicines created out of the earth which a wise man ought not abhor. Certainly, if one generally disapproves of synthetic drugs or artificial foods, one cannot condone the synthetic odor chemicals preferred by manufacturers only for the sake of reduced costs and higher profits and made for the commercial exploitation of emotional hedonic responses, or to produce behavioral modification with short-sighted goals and superficial or deleterious results. A purpose of authentic aromatherapy is to maintain or restore healthy, natural olfactory and psychological responses and to promote genuine, enduring self-improvement through the use of essential oils. Whole, pure essential oils, like whole foods, are better received by the human organism; they are more psycho-physiologically nourishing, carrying complete, intelligent information and messages to the human being. Their effects are not superficially stimulating but are safely therapeutic and capable of engendering real and profound changes. The subtle subjectivity of individualized smell and the complexity of essential oils may be too inconvenient or complicated for the consideration or objectives of medical establishment and fragrance industry practices, but they remain as necessarily vital to aromatherapy as they are personally important to the individual human being. Socialized environmental fragrancing is not aromatherapy. Mass aromatherapy of any kind, by practice or production, contradicts holistic individualized treatment and personal self-improvement—the purpose of aromatherapy's "individualized prescription" as declared by Marguerite Maury.

Modern man is in olfactory recession partly because of the evolution of other, more advanced senses but also because we are saturated and desensitized by the odorous stimuli of a more complex world and existence. Since we are already besieged by countless odors, scents, fragrances, perfumes, and aromas, there is reason to be more selective or more prohibitive with deliberate environmental fragrancing by still more synthetic aromatic substances. (We cannot predict that real essential oils or otherwise natural scents will be used in environmental fragrancing; yet, for ethical and philosophic reasons we ought not to endorse such use.) What are the potentially adverse health effects of widespread environmental fragrancing? Despite the increased likelihood of sensitization, synthetic fragrances will probably be favored for their lower manufacturing costs, and because of the reproducibility and predictability of human response to the narrow spectrum of components in synthetic scents. Yet, synthetic odors are apt to exacerbate concerns over the dangers of "second-hand scents" and heighten the debate over natural versus artificial substances. Scents are everywhere—but what of increased scented packaging? Already the "chemically hypersensitive," or people with allergies, have successfully protested "scratch and sniff" advertising and perfumed magazines. Responding to one of environmental fragrancing's proposed objectives, one might ask how "sensory engineering" hopes to actually improve air quality by generating more synthetic, artificial odors, regardless of how aromatically pleasing they may be. We ought to expect that artificial scents bring artificial results that are transient and superficial. Always, the issue of environmental fragrancing carries both health and ethical implications, the latter a clash between indiscriminate collectivism versus individual needs, preferences, choice, and liberty.

Using natural scents to attain therapeutic psycho-physiological effects in medical offices, hospitals, nursing homes, spas, or wherever else they might be expected or personally desirable (as at home, where one retains individual controls) is quite different from having government authorities pump fragrances into subways in the hope of deterring urban crime. (Religious liturgical incense rituals are not a sure argument for public environmental fragrancing, because people in church presumably share a single, common mental and spiritual imperative and expectation and are willingly bound by a single, unifying spiritual purpose arrived at voluntarily.) As for business offices, it will no doubt be argued that environmental fragrancing is both an employee benefit as well as an employer's advantage. But in any case, or more specifically in public subways, schools, or even prisons, environmental fragrancing is nonetheless mass medication akin to the fluoridation of water. Modern medical practitioners and civic authorities have, for their own reasons, chosen to ignore the existing and mounting scientific evidence that fluoride ingestion from city water is hazardous and injurious, owing not only to fluoride dosage alone but also to fluoride's interaction with other chemicals also present in the treated water. What is the interaction of synthetic scents with other odorous (and odorless) chemicals already present and interacting in the air, which synthetic fragrances may mask but do not eliminate, detoxify, or disarm? Always vulnerable to the law of unintended consequences, good intentions are not enough. Otherwise, we'd pump antibiotics into the air and water during respiratory or other epidemics.

These are some of the topics for debate generated by the matter of environmental fragrancing, especially in a pluralistic society such as that in the United States. Voluntary, informed individual consent, which may allow much smaller group consensus, is the best answer. Of course, natural scent ingredients, preferably essential oils, should always be selected, whether by collective consensus or individual choice. Ideally, the desired goals must be articulated and the results demonstrated to the satisfaction of those involved. More likely, no matter how well intentioned, environmental fragrancing will meet resistance, much of it justified, as it expands too far, too fast.

In addressing the behavioral modification aspects of environmental fragrancing, it is instructive that the effects of those social olfaction experiments recounted earlier were neither unanimous, total, nor scientifically reliable, because so many other factors and stimuli were unaccounted for. As if other sensory mixing or intrusion into our smell appreciation were not complicated enough, human response to scents, fragrances, odors, and aromas has many peculiar psychological variables—learned association or experience, associated or cognitive expectation—as well as other sensory, environmental reinforcements. The psycho-physiological effects of odors are difficult to trace or differentiate because individual differences profoundly affect any therapeutic result, even as shown by olfactory research involving simple synthetic scents—all of which complicates any strictly biological explanation for the effect of smell, or scent, upon human behavior. Correspondingly, the power of mind over matter may obviate or allay some fears of a sinister "scent slavery" like that practiced by the predator ants upon their victims, just as the exercise of individual free will mitigates the supposed irresistibility of suggestion.

# 5

# Psychotherapeutic Effects of Essential Oils

The psychotherapeutic benefits of essential oils may be derived by inhalation (olfaction to the brain) as well as by blood-borne (physiological) transmission by ingestion or transdermal absorption. The psychoactive effects of an essential oil are, of course, determined by that oil's nature and the potency and immediacy of effects are determined somewhat by the method of application; e.g., sedative essential oils are psychoactive by ingestion but are more quickly effective, even at smaller doses, by inhalation. The absorption rate differences among the applied methods of aromatherapy allow for versatility and some tailoring of responses, say, to stimulant oils, whereby the effects can be made more gradual or rapid according to the situational requirement.

The psychoactive effects of essential oils are recordable by electroencephalogram (EEG) measurements showing brain-wave responses expressed in brain-wave amplitude and frequency. Odors produce cortical brain-wave (EEG) activity responses involving alpha, beta, delta, and theta waves. Earlier, we cited the experimental work of Professor Shizuo Torii and his colleagues at Toho University in Tokyo, showing how jasmine increases alertness and attention by stimulating beta brain-wave activity and the contingent negative variable as measured by CNV amplitude. The sedative characteristics of lavender were also demonstrated, measured by EEG and CNV amplitude. A few years ago, at the Twenty-second Japanese

Symposium on Taste and Smell, Dr. H. Sugano of the University of Occupational and Environmental Health in Kitakyushu, reported his university's findings affirming Torii's research on jasmine and lavender. Once again the arousing characteristics of jasmine were demonstrated, as were the normalizing, relaxing effects of lavender. Lavender increases restful, meditative states, alpha brain-wave activity, mental concentration, and cerebral blood circulation. Sugano reported too that alpha-pinene, a primary terpene constituent of Japanese pine needle oil that is also found in varying percentage amounts in other essential oils, did likewise. Alpha-pinene is the principal constituent of turpentine oils distilled from the oleoresin of several members of the Pinaceae (fir, pine, spruce, hemlock) family. Isolated by fractional distillation and further purification, it forms the basis for synthetic camphor and pine oils as well as synthetic commercial products. Dr. Sugano suggests that the results provided by alpha-pinene support the healthful practice of strolling in pine forests. Aromatherapists know that the restorative, refreshing effects of pine forests are carried by the essential oil of pine, which imparts bracing, strengthening, and stabilizing psychological effects.

In 1991, at the aforementioned Second International Conference on the Psychology of Perfume held at Warwick University, Tyler Lorig of Washington and Lee University, whose experiment with the subliminal effects of synthetic musk was also mentioned earlier, asserted upon his own experimentation that the differences in EEG, or brain-wave, responses to jasmine and lavender found by Torii, Sugano, and others are not necessarily indicative of direct psychoactivity by odor stimulus on the central nervous system but can also be the result of cognitive factors or expectations. This may be so, but Lorig's findings do not refute those of the Japanese studies or the actuality of direct action by essential oils or other odorants. Having discussed this matter earlier, we repeat: While there are indeed mediating cognitive expectations involved with the perception of odors, that alone does not disprove or preclude an odor's actual or correlative physiological effects or, in this case, real psychoactive effects not caused by mere association or suggestion. It may or may not be that the cognitive expectations are justified by learned associations, acquired by personal experience, or even genetically codified into the collective memory of the human species. Moreover, that cognitive expectations can produce like results, as Lorig claims, doesn't mean that cognition had any influence upon the Japanese studies. Meanwhile, the corroborating experimental and experiential evidence of the psycho-physiological effects of jasmine, lavender, and other essential oils is quite convincing.

At the Second Malaysian International Conference on Essential Oils and Aroma Chemicals, held December 3–5, 1990, in Kuala Lumpur, Professor Leopold Jirovetz of the University of Vienna, Austria, presented his own conclusive research evidence that lavender, by its direct action upon the central nervous system, dramatically reduces hyperagitation in mice caused by the injection of caffeine. Therefore, even if cognitive expectation did play a role in the Japanese studies, we nonetheless know that lavender has the sedative psychoactive capabilities demonstrated by Torii and Sugano and that the expectations of the human subjects, if not those of the mice, were rightly realized.

## HORMONES AND NEUROCHEMICALS

We have learned that essential oils known for their antidepressant, sedative, or tranquilizing characteristics trigger the release of endorphins and enkephalins (neurochemical analgesics and tranquilizers) and, by other studies of odorant effects upon mood, how they may also influence other endogenous opiates within the brain. Essential oils also signal the activity of the hypothalamus and of hormones secreted by the endocrine, or ductless, glands, so called because they have no tubes, ducts, or openings carrying their hormone secretions away but instead release them directly into the bloodstream. These hormones act upon different parts and junction points in the brain and may also concentrate in special neural cell areas from which they may also be released.

Most of the body's hormones are produced by the endocrine glands. The pineal and pituitary are in close proximity to each other, each attached to the base of the brain, located behind the root of the nose, and approximately in the center of the head. The two adrenal glands sit one atop each kidney. The thyroid is positioned at the base of the neck, virtually surrounding the windpipe just beneath the larynx; two pairs of parathyroid glands reside in or near the thyroid. The thymus is in the chest. The pancreas lies across and behind the stomach. The gonads—ovaries and testicles—are yet more glands, near which significant cells are located. Hormones regulate most if not all vital bodily processes. Every single body cell is influenced in some way by these chemical messengers.

It has been estimated that the average human cranium contains as many as 100 billion neuron cells, each the tiniest fraction of an inch in length and connected in a thousand or more ways with other neurons at gapped junctions called synapses. Nerve activity involves electrical signal transmissions within each neuron cell and chemical transmissions between neuron cells. A neuron's receiving system is composed of dendrites; its sending system is called an axon. Dendrites are a webbing of fine, delicate fibers meeting the axons of other neurons from which signals are sent and received across the synaptic gap. A receiving neuron's dendrites are stimulated by a sending neuron's chemical neurotransmitters, some fifty kinds of which are known. These neurotransmitters pour across the synaptic gap, finding specific receptors on the neuron located on the other side of the synapse. Once arrived, they trigger various reactions. Having done their job, the neurotransmitters are either enzymatically broken down by the receiving neuron or reabsorbed by the sender. The entire process occurs in a mere few thousandths of a second.

Ordinarily, a neuron works on an "all or nothing" principle: if it fires at all, it fires as hard as it can. A strong enough stimulus triggers the same neuron impulse of identical strength; a weak stimulus is otherwise ignored. Neurons obtain their electrical voltages from ion-charged particles common in body fluids. In a normal resting state, a neuron holds a negative electrical charge in relation to the positively charged surrounding fluids, from which the neuron and its fibers are shielded by a membrane. When a neuron fires, it permits the positive charge to enter. If the neurotransmitter signals are of sufficient power, the electrical potential of the receiver neuron changes, and the electrically converted signal is fired down its axon, where the neuron's own chemicals are released, sending the signal across yet another synapse. The process is perpetuated from neuron to neuron, across thousands of neurons simultaneously. Each second as you are reading this, more than 100,000 chemical reactions are occurring in your brain.

What has just been described is a very simplified rendition of what actually happens. Structurally and functionally, the brain is more astoundingly intricate than we are capable of knowing or explaining by all that has been written about it, much less by references to a few of its known neurochemicals or its basic anatomical features, especially since brain cells also operate by bioelectric codes and electric wave transmissions as well as by the plenitude of biochemicals produced by the body. To give some idea of the brain's immense operational power and activity: A computer having the same number of "bits" as the average human brain weighing three pounds would stand a hundred stories high and cover the state of Texas. Too, there is much we do not know and little we fully understand about the highly complex independent functions and interactivity of the endocrine glands.

Because of the complex biochemical nature and homeostatic intelligence of essential oils, the hormonal effects of essential oils cannot be neatly classified as "uppers" or "downers" (as are single-action drugs), and neither do the glands' natural hormones behave in such a simplistic fashion. Human hormones are transformational substances having to do with every conceivable aspect and developmental level of human consciousness, perception, and intelligence, involving psychological functions of awareness (thinking, feeling, sensation) and moods as well as biological functions such as metabolism and homeostasis. Carrying the phytohormones of the plant kingdom, essential oils serve as a complement to human hormones in all those ways.

It may be that "sedative" oils trigger serotonin (a pineal gland hormone) and that "stimulating" oils trigger noradrenaline (NAD, a precursor to adrenaline) secreted by the adrenals; but we ought not to base such inferences upon unsteady suppositions about the nature of hormones or essential oils. First, a simple dual classification of essential oils into sedative oils or stimulating oils has not been and cannot be categorically established. Terms like *sedative, tranquilizer,* and *stimulant* are too broad and vague to describe the essential oil hormonal effects upon the many mixed moods and psychological states that occur on the wide spectrum of human emotion. Extending beyond the opposite points of arousal and repose, these states and moods also vary qualitatively from subtle to intense and from positive to negative. Of course, all essential oils are stimulative in the sense that they act as stimuli, and often one essential oil may be able to trigger both serotonin and other hormones, since so many are normalizing oils. Too, we should not conclude that serotonin and NAD have narrow, finite capabilities or effects as do "uppers" and "downers." Neither should we assume that they (or their respective glands) are antagonists or the sole or even the primary operatives in the balance between extremes of excitation and composure. Other glands and their hormones are also actively involved, as are other body systems.

Serotonin and NAD are not the only hormones produced by their respective glands. The inner part of the adrenals, the adrenal medulla, produces NAD and adrenaline, which is six times stronger than noradrenaline alone. The outer part of the gland, the adrenal cortex, produces some 30 to 50 glucocorticoids, mineralocorticoids, and sex hormones, which have various sustained effects beyond the speedy arousal provided by adrenaline. These substances are known collectively as corticosteroids or steroids, chief among which are two glucocorticoids, cortisone and cortisol, or hydrocortisone, recognizable by association with the similarly named and widely used synthetic drugs. The adrenal glands may actually produce as many as 100 different substances, each in precise amounts required by the human organism.

It is instructive that synthetic hormones are single preparations, often not even found in nature, taken out of the context of more complex hormonal formulas and potentized completely out of natural balance. Because of this, and because it is impossible for any physician to predict the constant metabolic adjustments the human body makes in the course of one day and then fine-tune the appropriate dosage, the side-effects of synthetic hormones are both numerous and severe. Ironically, in the attempt to duplicate the action of natural hormones, synthetics actually mimic the activity of a gland or endocrine system gone haywire, which is exactly what happens as the synthetic hormone deranges the entire system and consequently everything else in turn. Cortisone medication administered by intramuscular or intravenous injection or especially orally is perhaps the most well-known example of this.

Cortisone was discovered in the adrenal secretion in 1936, isolated first as a pure compound, then later synthesized as a pure chemical. Cortisone or steroid medication (most commonly prednisone, but there are others) suppresses the function of the adrenals, which, after the treatment is discontinued, may take several weeks or perhaps several months to begin functioning again—that is, if they begin functioning at all; if not, the patient is left with iatrogenic Addison's disease, or hypoadrenalism. Causing the adrenals to permanently cease production condemns the patient to permanent cortisone drug "treatment"—i.e., steroid addiction or dependency. But what drugs will compensate for the absence of cortisol, deoxycortisol, corticosterone, deoxycortisterone, aldosterone, and the rest of the hormones the patient's adrenals can no longer make?

Besides adrenal atrophy, other known side-effects of synthetic steroid treatment (most commonly using prednisone) begin with weight gain from increased appetite and salt and water retention, the latter causing severe edema and hypertension (high blood pressure). Increased appetite, resulting from the physiological stresses of disturbed protein metabolism and accelerated, excessive depletion and/or excretion of many vital nutrients (vitamins and minerals), coincides with increased stomach acid and enzyme production, which causes dyspepsia and likely peptic or gastrointestinal ulcers. By disturbing calcium and bone metabolism, more specifically causing osteoporosis and avascular necrosis (the loss of blood supply to the bones), steroid treatment leads to easy or spontaneous bone fractures and skeletal collapse. Since steroid or cortisone treatment impairs natural immunity, killing phagocytes and mononuclear cells and shriveling the thymus and lymph glands, susceptibility to infection increases, and wounds heal badly and more slowly. Additional steroid treatment side-effects include spontaneous hemorrhaging; elevated cholesterol and hyperlipidemia; hyperglycemia and pancreatitis (diabetes); glaucoma; convulsions; and psychopathy or psychosis.

Many other internal and external factors or stresses (congenital, psychological, environmental, nutritional) can acutely or chronically disturb the endocrine glands, but normally they operate with delicate and intelligent precision, administering what is necessary in minute measure and amounts. Too little or too much hormone will produce adverse results. Indeed, too much adrenaline may produce effects the opposite of those expected, just as too much serotonin can allergically heighten agitation rather than soothe. Ordinarily, low levels of serotonin are associated with hostile, even violent, antisocial or criminal human behavior and also with hyperactivity and aggression in children. (Schizophrenics have unusually low levels of serotonin.) This and the rest of what has just been said here about the endocrine system should persuade you to cautiously examine general assumptions and inferences made about the nature and activity of essential oils and hormones.

For now, consider holistically that an essential oil's known affinity for or action upon a given gland (or any other organ) must be understood on an oil-by-oil basis (e.g., geranium, pine, angelica, rosemary, and thyme each act directly upon the adrenals, but in different ways) and should not be thought of as exclusive. Thyme also acts directly upon the central nervous system and the thymus gland, geranium acts upon the pancreas, and pine affects the pineal. Indeed, essential oils participate with the entire endocrine system in a naturally intelligent and correct—hence safely balancing and stabilizing—way that is consistent with the system's own efforts to create and maintain harmony. So far, we know too little about the oils and glands and their hormones to say precisely how they interact. All we know for certain is that they do.

## ESSENTIAL OILS AND THE BRAIN HEMISPHERES

The understanding that all odorants are not created equal, that beyond your like or dislike of an odorant it has its own effects, applies to essential oils as well as to other odorous or aromatic substances. The odor response of the left hemisphere of the brain, either by direct stimulus or more often by transference of information from the right hemisphere, makes odor identification possible and easier (by whatever degree we are capable of it) because the left brain commands the highly advanced discriminatory functions of rational thought, speech, and language. The less discriminate, emotional, or hedonic response of the right brain occurs according to the dichotomous principle of attraction/repulsion and all its different either/or choices, making no further identifying distinctions about the source, value, or nature of the odorant stimulus. Here, we are reminded of the many criteria, aspects, and factors to be considered in selecting an essential oil for aromatherapy, beginning with the nature, properties, and characteristics of the oil itself and including such things as gender differences (in psychophysiology, in scent preferences, etc.) and the proposed method of essential oil application. We also consider the intended purpose and results. We know that by their very nature all essential oils are not equal or the same in their psychotherapeutic effects. Psychoactively, they may appeal more to one or the other brain hemisphere or may serve to better harmonize the activities of the two. Essential oils stimulating the right brain evoke emotional phenomena, responses, or activities (feelings, memories, imaginings); those stimulating the left brain affect intellectual processes (mental concentration, reason, judgement, logic) and evoke thoughts or ideas. In each case, the quality, extent, and intensity of effect will depend upon the individual; the nature and strength of the oil; and the surrounding influences, circumstances, and conditions.

Consider that the essential oil's elicited brain responses may or may not be advantageous to the task or situation at hand despite being otherwise favorable to one's well-being. This is the obvious point of our discussion. Logically, the oil selected must fit the intended mood or suit the intended purpose to arrive at the expected psychotherapeutic results. If you desire to promote left-brain intellectual processes, you do not select an oil that foremost appeals to the right brain, and certainly not a sexually stimulating aromatic substance like the musk oil which proved mentally distracting to the subjects in Tyler Lorig's experiment. The musk was synthetic, but Lorig's participants would have fared no better with real musk, especially since the subliminal administration of the scent contributed to its undermining effects upon mental concentration. (As we have said, if cognizant of an odor's presence, your mind can mediate or compensate by increased effort, in which case, unless an odor is sufficiently unpleasant or repugnant to drive you out of the room—or "out of your mind"—you can usually work through it, albeit less efficiently, productively, or comfortably.)

Otherwise pleasant or innocuous natural or synthetic odorants may or may not improve your mood, behavior, or performance; but to maximize your prospects and results you must use essential oils, nature's optimal scents. By their natural design, essential oils, more so than any other natural scents, act to heterolaterally harmonize the brain hemispheres. Synthetic perfumes, fragrances, and aromas have no such ability; in fact, they tend to operate in reverse, causing some disarrangement of the CNS and the body's etheric, electromagnetic field, and thus contributing to regressive homolateral activity and behavior. Essential oils that are inclined to favor one brain hemisphere, and so shift the focus of consciousness to one side of the brain, may be inappropriate choices for a particular purpose, but they do not in any way impair brain function. Essential oils are, after all, eminently healthful, beneficial substances, although their favorable psychotherapeutic effects may vary in certain ways for certain reasons. Beyond a person's peculiar aversion or unique allergic sensitivity to a particular oil, it will not have adverse effects when intelligently used by inhalation or topically according to the rules of safe essential oil usage in the practice of aromatherapy.

The psychologically harmonizing effects of essential oils upon the brain and endocrine system contribute to the integration of human intelligence, consciousness, and the total personality. It is by and during such integration, achieved by whatever means, that truly creative ideation and imagination are generated, inspired concepts arriving within the brain from a higher level of consciousness physically transmitted by the hormones of endocrine glands (most notably the pineal and pituitary) and bioneurochemicals. This transmission simultaneously occurs etherically or electromagnetically as well. It is the rare person who attains such integration permanently, but essential oils can help us do so with more ease, frequency, and regularity.

## ESSENTIAL OILS AND PSYCHOTHERAPY

Modern research into the psychotherapeutic effects of essential oils began with the smell-test experiments conducted by Giovanni Gatti and Renato Cayola, a pair of Italian doctors who, in 1923, published their findings in an article entitled "The Action of Essences on the Nervous System." In it they specifically discuss the possibilities of applying sedative and stimulating plant essences to relieve, respectively, anxiety and depression. Gatti and Cayola did not actually treat or experiment upon people suffering from those psychological states; instead, they set out to identify sedative or stimulating essences by measuring pulse rate and cardiovascular and respiratory activity before and after the inhalation of each essence. The two doctors' recommended list of sedatives to relieve anxiety includes neroli (orange blossom), petitgrain (orange leaf), cedarwood, chamomile, melissa, and valerian. Curiously, the single antidepressant recommended is ylang ylang, which they also cited, without explanation, as an aphrodisiac.

In the 1970s and 1980s, another Italian researcher, Paolo Rovesti, advanced Gatti and Cayola's observations by citing clinical experimental studies made upon actual patients suffering from what Rovesti describes as "hysteria or psychic depression." Unlike his two predecessors, Rovesti actually practiced aromatherapy to treat psychological ills, preferring inhalation as his method of application, and essence blends rather than single essences because he observed them to be more pleasantly received by patients. Rovesti confirmed Gatti and Cayola's favorable opinion of ylang ylang as an antidepressant and further recommended jasmine, orange, sandalwood, lemon, and lemon verbena. For anxiety, he also listed petitgrain and neroli, adding bergamot, cypress, lavender, lime, marjoram, rose, and violet leaf.

Essential oils can, of course, be used to treat many psychological ills and disturbances other than simple or profound anxiety and depression, which are often catchall terms for a variety of emotional moods, states, and conditions. There are essential oil aphrodisiacs for hypoactive libido and problems of impotence or frigidity, and there are euphorics to engender good feelings of well-being or elation. Some essential oils (e.g., clary sage, jasmine, ylang ylang) are both.

## Aversion Therapy and Positive Reinforcement

We alluded earlier to clinical attempts to make use of pleasant odors to create positive reinforcement behavioral modification (e.g., the behavioral techniques of Dr. Susan Schiffman and experiments involving MRI or cancer patients). Despite the findings of Ehrlichman and Bastone indicating that unpleasant odors have more influence upon moods than do pleasant odors, it nonetheless seems that positive reinforcement using pleasurable scents is usually more productive, in the long term at least, if not more immediately effective than negative aversion therapy techniques using harsh odors such as ammonia. This is because pleasant odors are not rejected, physically or emotionally; hence they penetrate deeper into the psyche and the memory. Professor Paolo Rovesti, by his aromatherapy approach to psychological ailments, affirmed this more ancient therapeutic concept of using pleasant odors to heal the psyche. Olfactory response to odor stimulus, whether to an essential oil or some other odorant, is more effectively utilized when accompanied by a physical therapy (e.g., massage), learning practice, and/or cognitive intellectual exercise. This knowledge is applicable by standard psychotherapeutic procedures and behavioral modification techniques involving learning, conditioned reflex, and partial reinforcement.

## The Learning Formula

A *conditioned reflex* is one that through learning has become attached to a conditioned (or a previously neutral) stimulus. A key ingredient to conditioned reflex is *partial reinforcement*, to be provided on some but not all occasions. Simply stated, learning is most likely to occur when there exists (1) a distinctive stimulus, (2) attention to that stimulus, and (3) some previously learned behavior to which that stimulus can be associated. It is important that the stimulus be distinct, that it will attract attention, and that there be an absence or minimum of distraction—i.e., that the stimulus be overriding. This formula generates *interest*, which is the key to memory.

Psychologically, human beings respond in one of two ways: by *stimulus generalization*, having learned to associate a stimulus with a particular behavior, then displaying this behavior to similar stimuli, or by *stimulus discrimination*, making unique distinctions between stimuli that are similar but not identical. Human beings possess the highest capacity for both responses, but it is the higher level of stimulus discrimination that separates us from the rest of the animal kingdom. Olfaction, it must be remembered, is a more primitive sense linked to physical and emotional responses that are generalized rather than selectively discriminate. It is training by mental cognition that permits greater refinement of olfaction response to odors and toward a higher discriminatory function.

Aversion therapy and positive reinforcement using odors capitalizes on the *pleasure principle*, a psychological concept Freud borrowed from Plato that describes the primary orientation of life toward pleasure and away from pain. The primary physical and emotional functions of awareness (sensation and feeling) and their psycho-physiological perceptive systems, mechanisms, and responses are deeply connected to the fundamental pleasure principle, which is an imperative for intrinsic satisfaction—i.e., the attainment of good personal feelings. The psychosomatic intimacy of the emotional and physical features of human nature, and the fact that human beings tend to remember physical motor skills better and longer than intellectual verbal skills, are clues to the importance of physical therapy or practice and the essentiality of physical responses to learning and behavior modification techniques.

We are reminded, too, that smell operates by the rules of attraction/repulsion in serving the pleasure principle, directing the organism to avert pain and seek pleasure. Instinctively and by learned association, smell provides information about physical safety or danger, pleasantness or unpleasantness, and pursuit or avoidance, in survival matters involving sustenance and procreation. Human beings have evolved newer hedonic, aesthetic responses and needs, mixed into the fundamental functional responses and purposes of smell, which have both clouded and heightened our sensory appreciation of odors. The fragrance industry has already successfully exploited our sophisticated olfaction even while preparing to venture further by offering us "aroma-chology" and "behavioral fragrances" that imitate psychology and psychiatry's predilection for behavioral modification techniques.

In this we can once again see and compare the difference in objectives between authentic aromatherapy, the scientific medical establishment (psychiatry), and the fragrance industry, according to each's approach to the physical, emotional, mental, and spiritual features of human nature and consciousness, and by how each appeals to and utilizes that feature's perceptive and evaluating powers of awareness, judgement, and response. It is noteworthy that among them only aromatherapy offers an approach and appeal to the spiritual aspect of human nature.

No matter how effective "behavioral fragrances" and behavioral modification techniques employing conditioned reflex and exploiting the pleasure principle seem to be, they do not produce real or profound transformational change. No genuine or permanent self-improvement in one's character, abilities, perceptive intelligence, performance, or circumstances can be achieved unless one's conscious cognitive thoughts and willpower—not just one's psychosomatic feelings—are actively engaged and improved. Authentic aromatherapy's betterment of the psyche and body is in the interests of improving the mind and character—the entire individual—helping to integrate the total personality by harmonizing all features of human nature and consciousness. Aromatherapy does not merely elicit or instigate psycho-physiological responses or behavior modification, nor does it stimulate or promote transitory moods and "good feelings" apart from the higher mental and spiritual aspects and aspirations of human nature and consciousness.

# MEMORY

## Memory and Odors

Although the work of Ehrlichman and Bastone, and of Steve Van Toller at Warwick University, suggests that olfaction memory differs little in time of acquisition and forgetting compared with memory involving sight or hearing, their findings may not be entirely conclusive. Other studies indicate that long-term odor memory is stronger than long-term visual memory. This is partly because of our primitive, self-preservation or species-preservation instincts and most probably because the subconscious connections to smell use far less stimulus discrimination than does conscious sight. Hence, there is more inherent prejudice and irrationality in smell evaluations because they are more inclined to stimulus generalization. The physical and emotional features of human nature are slower to learn but also slower to forget, a fact that must be accounted for in any assessment of smell and odor memory. In any case, we do know that learned associative smell, as is employed in aversion therapy and positive reinforcement, leaves a lasting impression and that odors can be useful therapeutically to jolt or prompt recall, even in cases of amnesia or co-matose conditions. It does seem likely that the elephant's legendary and deserved reputation for long memory is due to its extraordinary reliance upon its long nose.

Presented in the July 1990 issue of the *Journal of Experimental Psychology: Learning, Memory and Cognition*, the work of researcher Frank Schab at Yale University provides what Brian Lyman of Monell Chemical Senses Center describes as the first firm scientific evidence that odors can help evoke memories. In his experiment, Schab, who has since conducted psychological research at the General Motors Research Labs in Warren, Michigan, demonstrated that college students who smelled chocolate during a word exercise, and again during testing the next day, remembered their answers better than did those who were not offered the scent. In one experiment using this smell-association memory exercise, seventy-two Yale undergraduates were presented a list of forty common adjectives and asked to write down an antonym for each. They were not informed of the plan to test their answer recall the next day. Some students were exposed to chocolate scent during the word-matching only, some during the later recall test only, some during both halves of the procedure, and others not at all. Schab added to the cognitive, intellectual exercise by asking every student to imagine the aroma of chocolate during both halves of the procedure. Those students actually exposed to the aroma during the entire procedure (word-match and recall test) recalled a measurably higher percentage of their answers (21 percent) than did the other groups, the best average from which was 17 percent. Significantly, a later experiment showed that the same odor must be present both at the learning and the testing to derive any memory association result. Schab suggests that a student studying for coincidental exams in different subjects could use a different odor cue for each. He also concludes that because chocolate aroma and the scent of mothballs worked equally well, the pleasantness of an odor does not alter its ability to stimulate recall; but that conclusion is not entirely correct and requires some examination.

First, the perceived pleasantness or unpleasantness of an odor is often a singularly subjective, personal opinion, the dichotomous evaluation of which depending greatly upon cognitive mediation and the odor's association to past or present events, circumstances, surroundings, and psychophysiological conditions. Moreover, the mere stimulation of recall adequately describes or addresses neither the nature, quality, value, or intensity of those memories recalled nor of the odorant used to recall them. By that criteria not all memories can be judged of equal worth, just as all odors are not created equal. The differences among them are less apparent when simple or inferior scents are used and compared, such as chocolate and mothballs, by which the students' improved performance, while statistically representable, was not particularly remarkable. Real differences among odors and the importance of scent selection become more dramatically significant when superior complex fragrances—essential oils—are introduced into the equation and process.

The concept and functional exercise of memory involves more than the temporary or permanent, planned or incidental provocation of recall. It includes the expansion of memory itself—the increasing capacity to remember and to do so independently upon personal mental command—and the improvement of human intelligence. By innervating the brain—indeed, the entire central nervous system—the essential oils of basil, peppermint, and rosemary, as examples, have the capability to stimulate not just recall but the mental powers of memorization and concentration. (It is not merely fortuitous that the word *mint*, as in *peppermint* or *spearmint*, shares etymological roots with the word *mind*.) Essential oils evoke and enhance intellectual, emotional, and physical functions of awareness and judiciary powers, according to whatever connection is made by an oil's nature to a respective feature of human nature or consciousness and its corresponding anatomical locations in the brain and elsewhere in the body.

## Mapping the Mind and Memory

Today's most widely accepted neurological theory was first conceived in 1937. The Papez-MacLean theory emphasizes the importance of the limbic system as a set of interconnected pathways in the brain related to the hypothalamus, the hippocampus, and some primitive areas of the cerebrum having to do with smell, oral movements linked to feeding and primitive exploratory behavior, fundamental drives for survival, and emotional and visceral responses. The limbic system also contains the "pleasure center," stimulation of which serves to reinforce learning. Advancement of the Papez-MacLean theory has since led to the limbic system's identification with memory. In tandem with the hippocampus it forms the central switchboard coordinating all sensory input into a coherent whole.

Only during the past few years have scientists been able to actually "view" human thought and memory processes, tracing the complex patterns of electrical and chemical reactions to certain areas and features of the brain. For example, an electronic imaging, "charge-coupled" device—a special, highly sensitive camera—can record small, subtle, otherwise invisible differences in reflected light flickering across the surface of the brain as thoughts occur, thereby allowing scientists to track those thoughts to specific brain locations. Likewise, by using advanced imaging technology known as positron emission tomography, or PET scanning, which is capable of making biochemical processes visible, researchers in 1991 photographed the memory formation process for the first time, providing not only confirmation of some previously held beliefs about the limbic system, hippocampus, and memory, but a few surprises as well.

## The Hippocampus

Located deep within the brain, behind the eyes and between the ears, the hippocampus is alternately described as a banana-shaped organ or a set of seahorse-shaped structures curling under like antlers on each side of the head. It pulsates a mysterious theta brain-wave rhythm that signals its functioning in modifying emotion and processing memory. (Recorded by EEG, theta waves provide an important clue to olfaction responses and effects.) The role of the hippocampus and limbic system in processing memory has previously been inferred from behavioral studies of people suffering from accidental or alcoholic damage to those regions of the brain. Such people suffer a complete loss of recent memory and a failure to newly memorize even the simplest things. Head trauma, especially, disrupts the hippocampus, resulting in memory loss that although sometimes retrospectively extensive is still more recent, usually leaving memories from childhood and adolescence intact. This provides the first clue that the hippocampus has a primary role in processing events and experiences into memories, but it is neither the sole processing point nor the final repository of long-term memory. Memory processing and storage also occur elsewhere in previously unsuspected areas of the brain.

As a particular kind of sensory stimulus repeatedly enters the same area of the brain, whole collections of neurons align into assemblies that mutually stimulate into similar and increasingly more reliable patterns, depending upon the continual stimulus reinforcement. This is what makes memory initially possible, providing what scientists call long-term potentiation or LTP. But because the brain records different stimuli in different locations—e.g., sounds in the auditory cortex, images in the visual cortex—it is the important central switchboard of the limbic system and hippocampus that must connect and coordinate them into a single, coherent whole. In this process, the hippocampus serves as a kind of way station in which memories linger for an extended but indeterminate period of time in a suspended state between short-term and long-term memory.

## PET Scanning the Brain

The brain regions undergoing the most activity typically require a larger amount of glucose from the blood; hence blood flow is increased in those brain areas. (Notably, less glucose used more efficiently is associated with superior intelligence.) By following a radioactive isotope of oxygen placed in a tiny amount of water injected into the bloodstream, the PET scan monitors the blood circulation carrying the needed glucose supply.

Using PET scanning, University of California at San Diego neuroscientist Larry Squire and Washington University neurologist Marcus Raichle studied eighteen healthy volunteer subjects to whom they showed fifteen multiletter words on a computer screen. Afterward, the same volunteers were shown a list of the first three letters of words (not all of which appeared on the initial list of fifteen), to which they were asked to respond by saying the first word that came into their minds or to attempt recall of any specific word from the initial list. When monitored forming new memories during the initial word learning experience, most of the subjects' brain activity (blood flow) was in the hippocampus. But when they attempted to recall specific words seen before, activity appeared not only in the hippocampus but also in the frontal cortex or lobes of the brain having to do with thought processes. Moreover, when asked not to recall specific words but only to say the first word that occurred to mind, brain activity occurred in the rear cortex region, at the back of the brain, known to be a processing center for visual informational input and the place where unconscious visual memory traces are left for a time before being dismissed or committed to longer-term memory by reinforcement. As expected, repeated informational input reduces the time and energy required for the brain to recognize the input (a picture, a word, etc.) upon each subsequent exposure.

Clearly, memory is a far more complex process involving far more of the brain than scientists once thought. But then there are different types of memories. It is important to realize that odor or smell memory does not necessarily engage other brain areas involved in the memory process unless smell occurs coincidental with auditory, visual, or thought stimuli and processes. The more it coincides, the more likely it is to be remembered, retained in the short-to-long term memory complex starting at the LTP cellular level and processed first through the limbic system and hippocampus.

Just as the rings in a tree tell its history, the layered folds and features of the brain represent a history of human evolution, beginning from a serpentine spinal cord to which is added a rudimentary brain stem and then brain centers for smell, body function control, primitive emotions, and so on. As the human organism became more complexly advanced, extending itself beyond the narrow confines of survival existence in which touch, taste, and smell are the earliest and preeminent senses, new superior brain features correspondingly evolved over the primitive "old brain" structures, developing and heightening both old and newly advanced senses, and modifying instincts and emotions by the development of mind. This brain development also created a larger memory storage capacity, expanding to accommodate everything in the extraordinarily vast human experience from food and foraging knowledge, gathered by man's wide-ranging behavior and omnivorous diet, to complex physical and mental skills and ingenuity, achievements, and accomplishments of inventiveness and creativity unsurpassed by any other earthly species.

Drs. Samuel Weiss and Brent Reynolds of the University of Calgary Faculty of Medicine have discovered in the brain tissue of adult mice a reservoir of immature cells that, when properly stimulated by a certain protein, show the potential to produce new nerve cells. Their research may yet prove that an adult mammal has the resources to produce new brain cells. Meanwhile, we are told that all the nerve cells of a healthy human brain exist at birth; the total number of neurons never increases. Yet, the brain grows in size and weight from eleven ounces at birth to nearly three pounds in adulthood, adding mass by developing neuron sheaths and including non-neuron supporting cells that develop in the brain after birth. Also, most importantly, mass is added by the growth of the neurons themselves, which can develop new dendrites just as a tree grows new branches. This growth and the increased production of neurotransmitter chemicals, such as acetyl-choline, is stimulated by learning.

# METAPHYSICAL OBSERVATIONS

## Memory and Interest

As an explanation for memory processes, psychology has postulated the existence of *engrams*—otherwise undefined impressions or memory traces made upon protoplasm, the "stuff of life." In reality, it is upon ether, the true stuff of life, that these enigmatic engrams are actually impressed: into the etheric protoplasm of the etheric double and, to a lesser extent, the astral body. An etheric engram serves as a mediational mark often visible to psychic sight (and perhaps someday to Kirlian photography or other technology) as an image, symbol, or shape within the human aura. When memory traces aggregate and persist, so too does memory; when they are washed out, the person forgets. Memory traces cluster by the power of attraction—the major operating force within the astral plane, where like attracts like. The other operating force is repulsion, attraction/repulsion being the dichotomous evaluating principle in the function of feeling or emotion. The idea that we attract what we are derives from the astral plane or level of consciousness. The concept that opposites attract applies principally in the material world of dense, physical matter and appearances.

To say that memory is interest is to say that it is influenced by suitability. In the estimation of William James, this is a function of consciousness, "the selective industry of mind." Consciousness shows interest and attention by utilizing its selective, discriminative powers of mind to suit itself, remembering what it considers vital and rejecting what it sees as unimportant. Personal consciousness is the difference between human beings; each person scrutinizes information and learning situations in different ways according to personal interests and motives. If the subject matter can be made genuinely significant to a person's motivations, his or her attention, performance, and memory will heighten, and learning will improve. The degree to which memory engrams persist will depend upon (1) the human nature or consciousness of the individual, (2) the method by which a learning experience or behavior is introduced to that individual, and (3) whether the learned ability best suits that individual's nature—i.e., whether it can be shown to be of value and therefore of real interest to the individual. Learning, as James correctly discerned, is accumulative: the more you learn, the more you are capable of learning, and the more you will want to learn. This accumulation is like metal filings aligning together along invisible currents of electromagnetic force, just as physical neurons assemble themselves into patterns, and can be envisioned as etheric threads of knowledge being gradually woven into the fabric of an expanding intelligence, even as memories are woven into the fabric of our etheric being, visible as the aura.

## Thymos and Psyche: The Etheric Double and the Astral Body

The Greek word *psyche* describes what is otherwise referred to as the soul or astral body. The Greek word *thymos* distinguishes the etheric double that vitalizes and animates the dense, physical body (Greek: *soma*), providing the body its energy and motility. Unlike the astral body, which is composed of finer astral material, the etheric double is part of the physical world, generating the electromagnetic characteristics associated with the physical body. Both the etheric double and the astral body surround and interpenetrate the physical body; but whereas the astral body has an ovoid shape that extends to various distances from the physical body, the etheric double shares the contour shape of the physical vehicle and is in much closer proximity, extending beyond the periphery of the physical form as little as an inch or two. Belonging to physical existence, the etheric double is mortal, disintegrating soon after death of the physical body—usually in a matter of days. Conversely, the astral body is an independently separate vehicle that survives physical death; hence it is designated as the soul, owing to its greater longevity.

The etheric double (sometimes called the vital body) and the astral body are primarily the source of the phenomenon known as the aura. They are jointly responsible for the sensate and feeling responses, functions, and faculties of human nature or consciousness that are respectively differentiated as physical and emotional but which are deeply intertwined. That is, they are psychosomatic. The physical body and its etheric double determine physical sensation, instinct, primordial drives, and the biological emotions; the astral body governs the human feelings and emotional motivations (desires, passions), aesthetic motivational needs, and imagination.

## Mind and the Fourfold Human Nature

The Greek word *menos* describes the feature of human consciousness we call mind, which uniquely defines man. *Menos* means "mind/spirit," because the mind is closest to pure spirit in quality, function, and proximity. Life spirit, or causal spirit, is the highest element of human consciousness, of the fourfold human nature. A simplified outline of that nature is offered below; although sketchy, it is adequate for the purpose of our discussion.

| NATURE | VEHICLE | AWARENESS | MOTIVATIONAL NEEDS | CONSCIOUSNESS |
|--------|---------|-----------|--------------------|---------------|
| Spirit | Causal body | Intuition | Inspirational/Moral | Superconscious |
| Mind (*menos*) | Mental body | Thought | Intellectual/Mental | Conscious |
| Soul (*psyche*) | Astral body | Feeling | Emotional/Aesthetic | Subconscious |
| Body (*soma*) | Physical body | Sensation | Physical/Practical | Subconscious |

(*Note*: The etheric double (*thymos*) is not represented because it is part of the physical body and not an independently separate vehicle. Also, subconscious and superconscious features, although quite distinct, are more generally grouped as unconscious features because they exist outside the cognizance or perception of the conscious mind. Certain aspects of the body (*soma*) are actually preconscious rather than simply subconscious—a meaningful difference that, regrettably, we cannot digress to explain.)

All four features operate interactively and also function independently. The mind is, of course, responsible for generating thoughts and ideas, just as the psyche generates feelings and imagery, but each communicates with spirit and the body as well as with each other. For example, mind receives and imparts the superconscious impulses of spirit as creative ideas (ideation) in the left hemisphere; the psyche does likewise, but instead as creative images (imagination) arriving in the right hemisphere. Moreover, when it hearkens to the higher incentives of spirit, the psyche demonstrates the soulful behavior of spiritual love (Greek: *agape*) and unselfish devotion, and the love of beauty (aestheticism) as well as creative imagination. By contrast, when the psyche generates its own astral urgings or responds to the etheric physical impulses of the body, it demonstrates the more common romantic, hedonistic, and erotic behaviors of physical love (Greek: *eros*) and more personal or selfish emotional passions and desires.

As delineated, the mind has a clearer, more direct, and more immediate communication with spirit and thereby with intuition and the superconscious. Conversely, the mind, while relatively intimate with the moods and feelings of the psyche, is more distant and detached from the physical body and its needs, functions, and awareness. As a separate vehicle, the mind operates consciously and rationally. The physical body, like the psyche, is functionally subconscious and irrational.

## Genius and Intelligence

It should be understood that the human brain, left and right hemispheres, is the continually developing physical instrument and not the source or origin of the mind and psyche. There is far more to spirit, mind, and soul than can be contained or found in the human brain. Also, the greatest creative thoughts and ingenious ideas arrive to the left brain not from the right-brain psyche but rather from a higher, intuitive spiritual source acting upon centers in the head located proximately to the pituitary and pineal glands. Therefore, such great thoughts and ideas are charged not with emotion but with the dispassionate enthusiasm and inspirational genius of spirit. The so-called "spiritual centers" located in and at the cranium are the same generators that project to the psyche, which owing to the peculiar and less compatible construction of the right brain, receives such transmissions as creative images or imagination. Not only in different ways but for different purposes, the mind and psyche invite and are transformed by pure spirit, which transmits its urgings via physical and supraphysical instruments (organs and centers) that provide supraphysical, extrasensory perception and the superconscious, intuitive element of human nature and consciousness. If correctly and strongly focalized by the mind and psyche, spirit will activate these specifically located instruments to raise human intelligence and consciousness.

## The Etheric Nature of Plants and Essential Oils

It has been said that a plant's essence is its "soul," but this is meant only metaphorically. In reality, when we refer to a plant's essence, *soul* is a misnomer, because a plant has no astral body (hence no psyche or real soul) or any of the attendant or corresponding functions, responses, or capabilities of an astral nature. A plant's essence is made from etheric substance and fashioned by etheric force, which is the actual source of a plant's aura. A plant's essence, its vital body, absorbs and stores life spirit, principally from the sun (vital solar energy), in some ways similar to how the human etheric double does so. Since humans and plants exist on quite different levels of the evolutionary scale, there are of course enormous differences in etheric complexity, but the analogy is apt as far as it goes. Obviously, too, a human being has a mind, a greater spiritual capacity, and an astral body (psyche, soul) that provide superior motility, consciousness, intelligence, and sentience. A plant's unconscious existence roughly corresponds to a person's consciousness during deep, dreamless sleep.

The metaphorical reference to a plant's essence as its "soul," although inaccurate, is nonetheless useful. First, in the separate existence of plant life (not compared to that of man or animal) a plant's etheric essence is for all intents and purposes its soulful nature, illustrating how within plant life and activity, essential oils function according to the astral-etheric principle of attraction/repulsion, and also showing how essential oils cooperate with human nature by the principle of affinity.

As the expression or distillation of a plant's etheric essence, an essential oil has two basic functions: to attract certain animals, insects, and other creatures that promote the plant's health and propagation (fertilization), and to repel certain disease microbes and animal or insect predators, that harm the plant. The soul of a healthy, hearty person morally and aesthetically attracts good and rejects bad or evil. So, too, a healthy, hearty plant, by its etheric essence, vital body, or "soul" does likewise on its physical level of existence. It does this biochemically and electromagnetically (etherically) by the dichotomous principle of attraction/repulsion. Astral-etheric attraction operates by centripetal force; repulsion operates by centrifugal force. Respectively translated into scientific terms, these are the magnetic and electrical forces of positive/negative electromagnetism operating in the physical world. The electromagnetic/etheric charge of a plant's vital essence or essential oil acts physically and etherically at atomic, molecular, and cellular levels within humans and animals or otherwise for the plant's own purposes, which include its internal processes because essential oils are also a plant's hormones, containing biochemicals necessary to its own internal communication.

## Essential Oils and the Principle of Affinity

Affinity is a variation of the natural law or principle of correspondences or similarity. Affinity enables essential oils to act directly upon the psycho-physiologic features of human nature. Essential oils have biochemical, electromagnetic, and hormonal properties usefully similar and highly compatible to human nature and to human substances produced in the etheric and physical body: chemical to chemical, charge to charge, phytohormone to human hormone. This should hardly be surprising since our physical existence directly depends in various ways upon the plant kingdom. But essential oils have a contribution to make to our existence beyond basic survival. By its etheric substance, the essence of a plant, extracted in its essential oil, promotes memory. An essential oil's fragrant nature, with its volatile or lingering fumes, not only acts as a superior limbic-hippocampal stimulant but is actually absorbed into the human etheric double, assisting the aggregate formation of engrams. By their highly desirable compatibility, essential oils can promote interest: the key factor in learning and memory processes. Interest is what triggers the forces of attraction/repulsion and establishes affinity, whereby like attracts like. The inhaled effect of essential oils upon memory is even more pronounced when the oils are applied topically.

Unlike naturally inorganic or man-made synthetic substances, materials, and products, essential oils are very much alive. Unlike isolated constituents, essential oils are correctly and completely balanced in all their vital activity. Compared with other natural organic substances, plant essential oils are more healthful, vitally pure, and active. The psychotherapeutic activity of essential oils is at once biochemical-hormonal and electromagnetic-etheric, just as their physiotherapeutic nature acts simultaneously upon the physical body and its etheric double. Therefore, essential oils are psychoactive not only by their hormonal and biochemical effects upon the body and brain but also by their direct action upon the etheric double and reciprocally upon the astral body. The etheric double responds to the topical application of essential oils in the same way it does to their fragrance, which is why many traditional holistic health and spiritual practices involve the use of aromatic oils and unguents, to protect the etheric double and physical body from unwanted, unhealthful invasions and influences. Essential oils shield and invigorate the etheric double, magnifying the body aura by transfer of their own vital energy.

164

Traditional religious practices of ceremonial unction, or anointing with oil, continue to the time of death (as in the rite of extreme unction) and afterward to anneal the etheric double, sealing it from malevolent psychic (astral) intrusions and extending its life by slowing its disintegration, even as the material decay of the physical body is simultaneously retarded. This is done to ease transition and aid the passage of the soul. To an even greater extent than in liturgical services or religious gatherings, aromatics can be individually employed to promote spiritual rapture and personal meditation. For many centuries, Eastern and Western mystics and masters have done so to advance their spiritual and mental development and to improve the strength and quality of their auras. The most holy, like the Christ or the Buddha, by their spiritual and mental excellence and their purity of body and soul, generate their own sublime scent, which exceeds that of any earthly fragrance and imbues an indescribably magnificent aura that extends its power, heat, and light for great distances.

Essential oils act metaphysically, as well as physically, to harmonize and develop the fourfold human nature, most particularly via the physical, vital, and astral bodies.

# 6

# The Chemistry of Essential Oils

Historically, it was J. J. Houton de la Billardiere who conducted the first significant elementary investigation of the chemistry of essential oils by analyzing the oldest one known: oil of turpentine. His results, published in the early nineteenth century, revealed turpentine's ratio of carbon to hydrogen to be 5:8, the same (as later analyses would show) for all hemiterpenes, terpenes, sesquiterpenes, and polyterpenes. Terpenes, hydrocarbons abundantly found in plants, are clearly divisible by branched $C_5$ chains and are so classified as hemiterpenes ($C_5$), monoterpenes ($C_{10}$), sesquiterpenes ($C_{15}$), diterpenes ($C_{20}$), triterpenes ($C_{30}$), tetraterpenes ($C_{40}$), to all polyterpenes having any higher number of carbon atoms. Monoterpenes, sesquiterpenes, and diterpenes are particularly plentiful in essential oils, which also contain other chemical constituents such as esters, alcohols, phenols, aldehydes, and ketones.

Subsequent investigations and experiments done by the most notable nineteenth-century European chemists focused on the hydrocarbons contained in essential oils. Apparently the word *terpene* was coined in 1866. This active and expansive research paralleled the increased use of essential oils during the late 1800s, but it was specifically the research and development of terpenes and terpene derivatives that spawned the new essential oil industry that emerged at the start of the twentieth century. The molecular structure and chemical components of essential oils were then rapidly explored and identified, and these new constituents were synthesized and then commercially manufactured. The industry for synthetics and isolated

166

aromatics was born and with it a stark pharmacological perspective of essential oils that would have lingering ramifications in aromatherapy.

# CHEMOTYPES

The controversial theory of chemotypes can be considered a more recent offspring of the growth of chemistry that began in earnest some hundred years ago and that shares chemistry's urge to isolate or emphasize individual components of essential oils. Apparently, diverse growing conditions of soil and climate are frequently responsible for naturally produced ratio deviations in the chemical composition of plants that are otherwise botanically alike. These seasonal deviations are produced during the growth process and take place within the plant, not within the chemist's lab or the production process of the plant's essential oil. We have seen that the chemical compositions of thyme, rosemary, geranium, and other essential oils sometimes vary dramatically. Why chemotypes of a few plants emerge is not fully understood. They are found in the wild only as individual plants among a population having a mix of different chemotypes but sometimes one that, at least temporarily, predominates. Today, growers try to isolate and cultivate plants that have chemical compositions different from the expected norm of the plant, despite being from the same species, through extensive selection processes and restrictive growing procedures that sometimes include cloning. Advocates of chemotyping, such as chemist Pierre Franchomme, propose growing a particular species of plant in a certain soil and climate conditions or at higher altitudes to manipulate the oil's chemical structure. Chemotypes of thyme, rosemary, and eucalyptus are among a few deliberately obtained in these ways.

The concept of chemotyping plainly displays a kind of pharmacological viewpoint reflecting chemistry's inclination to utilize more of a specific chemical found within the oil or plant rather than the complete material or plant itself. Advocates of chemotyping within aromatherapy are presumably more comfortable with that idea because the desired chemical component is accentuated more naturally. Perhaps they do not fully consider that chemotyping is somewhat incongruous with the traditionally holistic inclinations and activities of aromatherapy and essential oils. Notwithstanding the worthwhile and important information that chemotype research provides, divergent opinions doubt the wisdom and value of strictly characterizing and prescribing essential oils according to their

167

alleged chemotype classifications. They cite the dangers of similarly repeating the errors in judgment, if not in actual practice, made by earlier
chemists whose zeal to isolate "active" ingredients or main constituents of
plants for the purpose of creating drugs instigated an imbalanced appraisal
of herbs and essential oils.

The eminent authority Dr. Jean Valnet recognizes a relationship between
the bactericidal power of aromatic essences and their chemical function,
beginning in descending order of potency with phenols, aldehydes, alcohols, esters, and acids. (There are differing opinions of the worth of terpenes, as we shall see.) He does not, however, specifically indicate chemo
types, emphasizing instead that the whole natural essence is found to be
more active than its principal constituents. Even Dr. Daniel Penoel, another proponent of chemotyping, whose interest in aromatherapy began
in 1977 with his professional association with Pierre Franchomme, admits
that the determination of the therapeutic use of an essential oil simply
from an analysis of its major chemical constituents is not a simple matter.
Penoel acknowledges the oil's action of totality, which seemingly confines
the use of chemotypes to specific clinical or medical uses. Dr. Jean-Claude
Lapraz, who worked with Dr. Valnet, is unwilling to concede even that specialized or limited role for chemotypes.

## The Law of All or Nothing

By his "Law of All or Nothing," Dr. Lapraz reaffirms the holistic viewpoint
of essential oil use with some scientific observations refuting chemotypes:

1.  It is not one particular antiseptic property (constituent) that de-
    termines the bactericidal activity of an essential oil.
2.  Regardless of its chemotype composition, an essential oil, by its
    own unique character or nature, either is or is not effective
    against a germ.
3.  The activity (effectiveness) or inactivity (ineffectiveness) of an
    essential oil depends on its botanical species, never on the
    chemotype or the season in which it is harvested or extracted.

Lapraz notes, for example, that essential oil of savory will have its ability regardless of when the plant is harvested or whether it contains more
or less carvacrol (a phenol). In a more explicit example, an essential oil of

thyme chemotype geraniol can be effective against staphylococcus, whereas an essential oil of geranium also containing geraniol will have no micro-biological effect on the same germ even if the thyme contains 40 percent geraniol or the geranium contains 80 percent geraniol.

The theory of chemotypes offers an interesting but contracted appreci-ation of essential oils that is still severely handicapped by incomplete knowl-edge of the hundreds—perhaps thousands—of identified and as yet uniden-tified constituents contained within them. Dr. Taylor of the University of Texas at Austin (cited by Valnet in *The Practice of Aromatherapy*) states that essences present more new compounds than the chemists of the whole world could analyze in a thousand years. If his statement is true, that hand-icap is not likely to disappear any time soon. For now, aromatherapy wel-comes new chemical data about essential oils while continuing to rely upon empirical knowledge and professional observations. Attention to its botan-ical species remains a reliable guide to an essential oil's behavior, since there is more practical value in knowing an oil's biological activity than in know-ing its chemical composition. The whole of an essential oil is greater than the sum of its parts, especially since we don't know what all those parts are. How an oil behaves therapeutically is crucial and displays a better, safer, more accurate and complete indication of its proper use. Otherwise, any preference for chemotypes remains subjective and—as with wine—some-what like a matter of taste.

## SAFE USE OF ESSENTIAL OILS

Another topic of some debate, involving both essential oil chemistry and quality, is safe use of essential oils—specifically, precautions and contra-indications. In this discussion, a sense of relative proportion ought to be established and maintained that first observes how few of the some 400 es-sential oils produced in the world pose any potential risks: the highest es-timates are between 10 and 15 percent. Considering that only 100 to 150 of those oils are used in aromatherapy worldwide, and that most toxic oils have never been commonly used, the risks dwindle even further. Nearly all of those hundred or so essential oils are available in Europe, where most are produced. Comparatively few, generally peppermint, spearmint, citrus, pine, and cedarwood oils, are produced in the United States. The U.S. Food and Drug Administration (FDA) lists approximately 150 oils for safe use in foods; about 100 essential oils are commercially extracted for sale to the perfume and flavor industries.

Although naturally derived, essential oils are highly concentrated substances with strong biological and chemical activities. However, it is important that while asserting their profound efficacy we do not overstate their possible hazards. A person runs a greater risk from using synthetic, spurious, or tainted oils than from using the pure essential oils of aromatherapy. Categorically, potentially hazardous oils may produce symptoms in three ways:

> *Toxicity*      (usually by ingestion and dependent upon dosage)
> *Sensitization* (allergic reactions arising from internal or external use)
> *Irritation*    (the least harmful reaction, usually resulting from topical application)

A few qualifying observations about essential oil use are worth noting. (1) As with any therapeutic treatment, children, pregnant women, and the elderly warrant additional precautionary considerations to avoid those negative reactions to which they are more susceptible. (2) Not all such oils are hazardous in all three ways; for example, a potentially toxic oil may be otherwise harmless when used topically. (3) Specific episodes of toxicity from essential oils invariably arise when the normal therapeutic dosage is greatly exceeded. Essential oil excretion from the body is typically so rapid and thorough that any harmful buildup would have to be caused by the excessive intake or application—or long-term use—of a specifically hazardous oil. It is important to our objective perspective that many overdose possibilities can and do result from ingesting natural and synthetic substances that are readily available and routinely acquired by the general public, not to mention the countless exposures to potential allergens and irritants— everything from household cleaners, pesticides, and cosmetics to drugs, alcohol, and apples. Ingestion of one cup of raw apple seeds is enough to induce death by cyanide released from within the seeds' natural amygdalin (vitamin $B_{17}$)—the same otherwise harmless and healthful nutrient found in almonds, apricot kernels, and many beans, peas, and seeds. There is no essential oil of apple seed. There is an essential oil of bitter almond used in flavoring after the deadly cyanide (prussic or hydrocyanic acid) has been removed. Bitter almond oil (not to be confused with sweet almond oil, a perfectly safe carrier oil for massage) is never used in aromatherapy. Incidentally, amygdalin from apricots is the active ingredient in Laetrile, a known cancer treatment. Apples and amygdalin illustrate how a natural nutrient can be converted into a healthful product or a harmful substance depending upon dosage and either foolish, correct, or intelligent use.

The particular hazard of an essential oil is sometimes, but not always, linked to its dominant constituent. Just as we may wrongly ascribe the therapeutic activity of an essential oil solely to one or two of its chemical components, we may also err in thinking that its risks are likewise attributable. Some potentially toxic or hazardous essential oils appear more often on cautionary lists than do others: wintergreen, pennyroyal, tansy, thuja, mugwort, mustard, savin, hyssop, wormwood, wormseed are a few. Others, such as cinnamon, anise, camphor, melissa, and fennel, appear intermittently, perhaps connoting an incomplete or inconclusive appreciation of whatever hazards or toxicity those oils may present. The inclusion of some oils predicated merely upon their chemical content—rosemary, sage, oregano, or thyme—is disputable, since there is little empirical evidence of their supposed dangers. Despite its thujone (a ketone) content, which is comparable to that of wormwood, tansy, and thuja, sage appears to be virtually risk free, probably because sage contains another unknown trace constituent or buffering agent that somehow prevents toxicity. Sage provides an important lesson in knowing the oil, not just its chemicals. Sage is sometimes contraindicated because of its hormonal properties, which stimulate the adrenals, but that is exceptional. This is true of other generally safe essential oils having hormonal properties, such as rosemary, thyme, savory, basil, geranium, cypress, fennel, and lemongrass.

Not just ketones, but phenols (which can be irritants) and terpenes, have been singled out as hazardous chemicals, and perhaps they may be when isolated or synthesized outside the plant. This does not necessarily make the oil that contains these constituents likewise hazardous. As drug manufacturing has shown, isolated ingredients from herbs are frequently made more hazardous as well as more potent. It is known that the possible toxicity of some food supplements (e.g., vitamin A, vitamin D, and iron) is far more likely from synthetic supplements than from natural vitamins and minerals. It is instructive that virtually none of the standard poisonous herbs, which are still obtainable, are aromatics.

Concern about chemical constituents in essential oils has led some people to deterpenization in an effort to eliminate the possibility of liver and renal toxicity from terpene-containing oils. It does seem untenable that hy-drocarbons like terpenes would exist so abundantly in plants and oils if nature thought them to be so inexpedient. Distrust of terpenes is seem-ingly unwarranted or at least exaggerated, since essential oils having the highest terpene content are among the least irritating. Some say that ter-penes are devoid of risks. Those who remain suspicious of terpenes argue that in any case deterpenated oils are safer while retaining their therapeu-tic powers and activities. This is not altogether true. A deterpenated oil is not complete. Deterpenating essences for aromatherapy lowers their bioac-tivity. Deterpenating thyme and bay leaf actually makes them more toxic or irritating, while deterpenating lavender—an oil already low in ter-penes—takes away its catalytic value.

The removal of any isolated ingredient from an essential oil used in aromatherapy does some injustice to the holistic action of that oil by im-balancing its properties and activities. Whereas the potential hazards of essential oils, particularly when given for internal use, are frequently over-stated, such real potentials are reduced or obviated by true aromather-apy practices. Inhalation and topical application present relatively minor risks of skin and mucous membrane irritation or temporary allergic reactions.

Regrettably, too many of those who warn of the potential dangers of es-sential oils, and advocate regulation and restriction of aromatherapy and essential oil use, have less than altruistic reasons for doing so. There are those in the aromatherapy profession and essential oil manufacturing busi-ness who desire to monopolize the practice and the sale of aromatherapy and its products. Some see an opportunity to achieve their ambitions by ingratiating themselves to government agencies and authorities, while oth-ers envision for themselves the kind of exclusive symbiotic relationship with the FDA now enjoyed by the pharmaceutical industry. Still others who favor restrictions and regulation are members of other health or medical professions who feel threatened by the competition of any new, successful health practice such as aromatherapy.

Manufacturers and distributors of vitamin and mineral supplements, health foods, herbs, and essential oils are prohibited from making specific health claims about their products, even though the health benefits of those products are well known and well documented. Otherwise, these food prod-ucts are exempt from the restrictions or regulations governing medicines and drugs. For this and other reasons, the FDA has no plans for regulating aromatherapy, despite urging from the would-be monopolists or jealous rivals. A claim that an aroma or fragrance is good or beneficial in a general way is classified as a cosmetic claim not requiring FDA approval before the product is sold. Only if an essential oil is marketed with labeling that specifically recommends it for treatment of an ailment, condition, or disease could it be subject to FDA approval.

Fortunately, there are many more conscientious aromatherapy practitioners and essential oil distributors and manufacturers who resolutely and objectively resist all self-interested efforts to control aromatherapy and its products. They rationally favor education for consumers, merchants, and practitioners that explains and emphasizes the facts and encourages intelligent, responsible use of essential oils and other aromatherapy products. Their concern for aromatherapy includes protecting the individual's rights and freedom of choice in health matters.

Like herbs and vitamin and mineral supplements, essential oils are foods, not drugs. Likewise, they should not be utilized indiscriminately. The wise health maxim "less is more" applies to aromatherapy. An otherwise safe and effective treatment for a given condition may actually worsen that condition if overused or overdosed. Minute doses of mugwort oil are used in homeopathy to treat convulsive disorders and epilepsy. In large doses it will cause convulsions. Qualified aromatherapists and phytotherapists know which essential oils to apply and which to avoid, and they always recommend small, precise dosages whether internally or externally. Consumers interested in using essential oils for their health or cosmetic benefits ought to be similarly educated.

# ESSENTIAL OIL ANALYSIS AND PRODUCTION METHODS

## Chromatography and Spectroscopy

Of those analysis methods used to characterize essential oils, gas chromatography (GC) is perhaps the most significant and the most controversial. A gas chromatogram of an essential oil is sometimes referred to as the oil's molecular "fingerprint," showing, for most authentic oils, from 20 to 50 (occasionally as many as 200) readily identifiable chemical constituents. Of course, any true quality evaluation of an essential oil should include all of its complementary secondary and trace constituents, which act synergetically upon the human body. Quality assessment or characterization of an essential oil solely by the percentage of an isolated or primary constituent, as is allowed by pharmaceutical requirements, is inadequate for aromatherapy. Such a simple criterion or characterization would permit a synthetic substitute having an acceptable level of one main ingredient to be falsely equated with a natural, more complex essential oil.

There are other chromatography methods: high performance liquid chromatography (HPLC), which uses pressurized liquids rather than gas and is especially effective for less pliable, hard to separate mixtures; gel liquid chromatography (GLC), a slower, less reliable and infrequently used method for essential oil analysis; and thin layer chromatography (TLC), which employs a thin layer of silica and is used more for the analyses of tinctures and extracts than for essential oils. Of these four, gas chromatography is the most common and effective.

Gas chromatography isolates different components of an essential oil, which appear as spikes or peaks in the chromatogram. The usefulness of this method strongly depends upon comparisons made with other chromatograms and standard reference material that only a specialized GC lab is likely to have. Still, it is difficult for the most expert analyst to know what to expect from an essential oil, since many plants, even the more familiar ones such as thyme, rosemary, and geranium, are constantly surprising researchers with newly found constituents and variable constituent ratios. Moreover, there are no universal standards for comparison. From which of as many as 100 different varieties of an essential oil do you select a standard model for comparison? Therefore, except in obvious cases of adulteration (usually with alcohol, fixed oils, essential oils of lesser value, or certain synthetics), analysis cannot be certain or conclusive.

To increase accuracy, mass spectrometry (MS) is sometimes combined with gas chromatography. Together, GC-MS provides a more valuable, albeit more expensive, analytical technique for essential oil research. There are other spectroscopic methods, such as infrared spectroscopy (using infrared light), ultraviolet spectroscopy (ultraviolet light), and nuclear magnetic resonance, but these are thought to be of little practical use to essential oil analysis. Mass spectrometry permits highly precise identification of chemical structures from molecules that have been shattered by high-energy electron bombardment. Generally, spectroscopy's value in identifying isolated components becomes severely limited when the method is applied to complex constituent analyses. As is so for chromatography, the interpretation of mass spectrum results is largely dependent upon the reference material available for comparison.

Given the high degree of technical skill and experience necessary to read a chromatogram (an interpretation that becomes even more complicated in GC-MS analysis) and the lack of reference data for which universal standards are nonexistent, chromatography, while contributing much to the elimination of synthetic compounds and pesticides in essential oils, alone has little capability of verifying an essential oil's purity. It may, in fact, by its ambiguity be misleading.

Although we must assume and respect the conscientious motives of those companies choosing to rely exclusively upon technology such as chromatography for quality assurance of their oils, we must also consider that such reliance is somewhat misplaced and premature, since technological essential oil analysis is hardly an exact science. Although gross adulterations are detectable, other factors cloud the issue of quality. First, sophisticated analysis methods have lent themselves to equally sophisticated adulteration techniques that can closely approximate the original "fingerprint" of the oil. Second, as alluded to earlier, new components are continually being disclosed even in long-studied oils—components probably indiscernible by chromatography. The percentages of those identifiable constituents often vary. One researcher found that the concentration of several recognizable chemical constituents in seven dozen species of thyme varied by as much as 50 percent. These variations are caused by the many factors (e.g., sun exposure, soil, geographical and botanical origin, time of year and extraction, and production process) that otherwise influence an essential oil's composition and so must be evaluated.

Most aromatherapy experts agree that essential oil production is much like wine making: more of an art than a science. Modern scientific olfaction research has increased our respect for the human sense of smell and has reemphasized the important role of an "educated nose" and its aesthetic sensibilities in the selection of good quality essential oils, as well as for the creation of essential oil blends for aromatherapy application. Most aromatherapists prefer to rely more on their own senses and their confidence in their essential oil suppliers. At least for now, the technological methods of analyzing essential oils have not produced results worth the high cost of equipment and operation.

## Continuous Steam Stripping

Steam distillation extracts an essential oil whose fragrance is as near as possible to that of the plant. Nonetheless, certain chemical reactions occur during the process that affect the chemical composition of the oil. Gradual improvements in manufacturing technology (such as modern still construction using steel to eliminate metal-to-oil reactions) and still design (a separate boiler to better control the temperature and pressure of steam generation) have likewise improved the quality of pure essential oils. Also important have been more recent variations in distillation, such as hydro-diffusion and turbo-distillation, each of which have increased essential oil yield in less time while retaining more of the plant's original fragrance. The latest and most promising steam distillation method, first attempted in 1981 by the Boucard Group, long-established essential oil distillers, and R. W. Serth, a chemical engineering professor at Texas A&I University, is Texarome's continuous steam stripping process. This method employs dry steam at temperatures often above 200°C to distill pulverized plant material for 25 to 30 seconds (called "residence time") at low pressure. It seems that the brief residence time prevents many of the chemical reactions that occur during normal steam distillation and, despite the high steam temperatures, is courteous to the natural chemistry of the oil produced. That the high steam temperatures apparently do not adversely affect the composition or fragrance of the oil is also attributable to the absence of air (oxygen) and moisture or liquid water in the dry steam process. This may also account for the reduced corrosion and erosion. The dry steam prohibits leaching of organic acids from the aromatic material that would not only corrode the apparatus but also catalytically affect the oil's chemistry. The steam stripping apparatus is designed to vaporize the entire liquid mixture instead of separating the mixture of compounds into fractions during the liquid phase, as occurs during traditional distillation. Hence, the operation is simplified through "stripping" of the entire liquid mixture from the inert plant material by low, partial pressure distillation.

## Supercritical Carbon Dioxide Extraction

We've already learned that the history of extraction began with the immersion of flowers and spices in fats and oil, particularly by the enfleurage method, which involves soaking plant material in a natural fat or mixture of animal and vegetable fats and oils. The plant material is then removed and replaced by new material each day for as long as a month. Afterward, the aromatic product may be treated with alcohol to create an "absolute of enfleurage" but is usually left as an aromatic oil. Why enfleurage has been almost completely abandoned should be obvious and unsurprising. True essential oils are now generally extracted by steam distillation and cold expression. Otherwise, solvents such as alcohol, benzene, or hexane are used for extraction, after which the solvent is removed by distillation, leaving a resinoid or concréte. Subsequently, the alcohol extraction of a concréte produces an absolute, from which the waxes and most of the solvent left in the concréte are removed. We know that the potential drawbacks of the elevated temperatures used in steam distillation methods are possible damage to the components of the essential oil and the loss of more highly volatile components. As for solvent extraction of concrétes and absolutes, we recognize that the residue of chemical solvents is practically impossible to remove completely. Today, carbon dioxide extraction is being hailed as the answer to these problems of high temperature and solvent extraction, because the temperatures used are relatively low and the only solvent, carbon dioxide ($CO_2$), in its gaseous state naturally evaporates or dissipates, leaving behind a pure plant extract. Therefore, carbon dioxide extraction is at least as clean a process as steam distillation, because similarly there are none of the residual solvents that might lead to toxicity either by themselves or from low-level contaminants within the solvent.

The carbon dioxide gas is brought to the supercritical state under certain conditions of temperature and pressure. The critical temperature of carbon dioxide is that above which it cannot be liquefied regardless of increased pressure. Its critical pressure is that below which $CO_2$ cannot be liquefied regardless of how low the temperature becomes. The supercritical state is attained when both temperature and pressure are above their respective critical points. Of low viscosity, supercritical $CO_2$ has the density of a liquid but diffuses like a gas. In this form it is capable of extracting into a solution the widest variety of constituents from the plant. In one case, for example, $CO_2$-extracted spearmint oil from field-dried leaves contained nine flavor components not acquired by steam distillation. Otherwise, supercritical $CO_2$ extracts are comparable in constituency to pure essential oils or concrétes.

It is after the supercritical $CO_2$ has been circulated through the plant material (located inside a special container placed within an extraction chamber), and has dissolved from it the desired fractions, that the then depressurized $CO_2$ becomes gaseous, loses its solvent capabilities, and separates from the created solution. The resultant solution of essential oil precipitates and is collected. The gaseous $CO_2$ is then released into a heat exchanger to be cooled, liquefied, and recirculated back to the extraction chamber under the same temperature and pressure conditions of the supercritical state.

A short summary of the factors recommending $CO_2$ extraction begins with the advantages it enjoys over steam distillation and solvents. The critical temperature (31°C) is low enough not to harm the delicate nature and properties of the plant's fragrance and essential oil. Besides leaving no $CO_2$ solvent residue in the extract, the process also does not extract any odorless resinous material. The critical pressure (73.8 bars) is easily attained in production operation; and carbon dioxide, which is commonly found in carbonated beverages such as soda pop and champagne, is known to be safe and harmless. Furthermore, essential oil extracts do not undergo the chemical reactions of oxidation, hydrolysis, esterification, or thermal changes and so remain more accurately representative of the original material. The primary disadvantage of supercritical carbon dioxide extraction is the high cost of production equipment and of the extraction operation, necessitating that the method be applied strictly to high-priced products. This might preclude the less expensive or low-yield essential oils that would not profitably compensate the high cost of their production. Indeed, there may not be enough profit in any large-scale carbon dioxide extraction of essential oils for aromatherapy purposes to redeem the expense of the process.

# 7

# Essential Oil Profiles

The following profiles are brief sketches of essential oils. These are abridged outlines of their more prominent features and are by no means a complete catalog of their properties, uses, or characteristics. Descriptions of their many clinical uses or applications for serious conditions are sparingly and only generally mentioned, since such treatments and ailments are better implemented and understood by qualified healthcare professionals. Although internal use of certain essential oils for therapeutic purposes can be inferred, it is not specifically recommended. Aromatherapy—inhalation and topical application—is emphasized. The profiles are intended to provide an introductory indication of the various ways aromatherapy and essential oils can be beneficial.

## ANGELICA (*ANGELICA ARCHANGELICA, A. OFFICINALIS, A. SYLVESTRIS*)

The essential oil is obtained from the roots or seeds. Angelica has carminative and stomachic properties that are helpful for a variety of digestive ills, including dyspepsia, flatulence, gastritis, and stomach ulcers. It is also indicated for hiccough and anorexia. A mild expectorant with anti-infectious qualities, angelica makes a useful inhalant or compress for lung ailments such as bronchitis and pneumonia, as well as for influenza. Its sudorific, antiseptic, and antimicrobial properties apply well in creams or lotions for skin ailments, although it may sometimes cause slight skin irritation.

Angelica's established reputation as a blood and lymph purifier derives principally from its ability to reduce excess uric acid levels in the blood, making it an especially valuable remedy for gout, rheumatism, and some forms of arthritis. Its blood cleansing activity eases circulation, thereby aiding the entire cardiovascular system.

Angelica stimulates estrogen production while also acting as an adrenal inhibitor that relaxes the nervous system. Its psychological effects are restorative and gently revitalizing, alleviating feelings of hopelessness and indecision as well as general conditions of nervous weakness.

# BASIL (*OCIMUM BASILICUM*)

Originally found in Asia, some 150 varieties of basil grow worldwide, many developing natural chemotypes. Common or sweet basil yields a light, greenish yellow oil (steam distilled from its leaves and flowering tops) having a delicious licorice-like aroma resembling that of fennel or tarragon. It is often used as a top note in modern perfumery. A popular condiment noted for its fine flavor and digestive benefits, basil is an intestinal antiseptic, carminative, and stomachic, indicated for various gastrointestinal ailments such as nausea and dyspepsia. As an inhalant, it is a valuable general treatment for respiratory ills, including asthma and bronchitis. In some cases, basil has been known to restore the sense of smell lost from rhinitis, sinusitis, or other causes. It is also good first aid for insect bites and stings. Basil's remarkable versatility makes it a favorite therapeutic agent in Ayurvedic medicine.

An emmenagogue and antispasmodic, basil is useful compress relief for menstrual pain. It contributes greatly to a relaxing bath. Combined with black pepper, for example, basil is an excellent massage treatment, assisting muscle tone and relieving fatigue. Basil also blends nicely with bergamot, geranium, hyssop, lavender, and rosemary for a variety of other applications. A natural nerve tonic, basil acts appropriately as a stimulant or restorative, depending upon the body's needs. Physiologically, basil's nervine properties effectually stimulate the sympathetic nerves and strengthen the adrenal cortex. Basil has cerebrospinal effects as well. It is therefore frequently recommended for numerous nervous afflictions, including epilepsy and paralysis. It relieves the symptoms of vertigo and fainting arising from varied causes, such as migraine headache. Basil is soporific (for insomnia) and antidepressant. Its versatility as a psychotherapeutic agent having homeostatic effects makes basil particularly valuable as a remedy for assorted psychological or psychosomatic complaints. It is a lively, revivifying antidote for melancholia and a good remedy for mental confusion. Basil eases the psychological discomfort of anxiety and apprehension or foreboding. It increases the body's radiant etheric energy, stimulates memory, and promotes mental clarity, acuity, and concentration. Basil's cephalic properties and activity are reminiscent of its Labiatae family relatives, peppermint and rosemary. Wrong use of basil may overstimulate body systems, causing nervousness or, inversely, stupefaction. Owing to its emmenagogic properties, basil is best avoided during pregnancy.

## BAY (*PIMENTA RACEMOSA, P. ACRIS*)

Essential oil of bay is steam distilled from the leaves of the bay tree, a tropical evergreen widely found in the West Indies. It has a strong spicy scent much like that of clove. Bay leaves distilled in rum is the traditional method and formula for producing original pure bay rum: an all-purpose tonic once used extensively for medicinal purposes. Today, a commercial "bay rum" is prepared for cosmetic use simply by adding bay oil to other oils in a mixture with alcohol and water. Cosmetic bay rum remains popular in the United States, the world's largest consumer of bay oil, which is also an ingredient in other perfume and fragrance industry products.

Genuine bay oil is a topical rubefacient used to increase scalp circulation and stimulate healthy hair growth; hence its inclusion in many shampoos and hair tonics, such as bay rum. Moreover, bay oil is antiseptic. Anti-infectious and decongestant, bay is recommended for respiratory ailments, for which it blends well with eucalyptus as an inhalant. Its analgesic properties are effective for rheumatic pain or neuralgia. Bay mixed with citrus oils or with spice oils are two of several combinations suggested for massage or a relaxing bath. Bay has a calming affect upon the autonomic nervous system. It may, however, cause mucous membrane irritation.

The ambiguity of the commercial designation "bay oil" to describe what may, in fact, be several different oils, creates confusion and underscores the importance of Latin names to properly identify specific botanicals. For example, the bay laurel ("sweet bay") evergreen tree or shrub found in the Mediterranean yields an essential oil steam distilled from its berries, leaves, and twigs. This bay laurel oil (*Laurus nobilis*) must not be confused with the bay oil from the West Indies bay tree (*P. racemosa* or *P. acris*). The bay laurel produces the bay leaves especially popular in French cuisine and as a beverage ingredient for its spicy flavor and odor reminiscent of cajeput. Bay laurel (bay leaves) is also a familiar fragrance component. Used as a digestive stimulant for congestive conditions and intestinal disturbances, bay laurel is carminative and emetic. It is also an emmenagogue, indicated for amenorrhea. Moreover, it is bactericidal, fungicidal, and a powerful insect repellent. Antirheumatic, laurel is likewise an effective treatment for sprains and bruises when applied in salves and liniments. Otherwise hypotensive and sedative, laurel has value as an antihysteric. It may cause some dermal irritation or sensitization (dermatitis) when applied topically, and it should be avoided during pregnancy.

(*Note:* to further emphasize the importance of Latin names and to anticipate any further confusion, it should be mentioned that pimenta oil, also known as allspice, is distilled from the berries or leaves of the pimenta tree [*Pimenta officinalis*]. It too is distinct from bay oil [*Pimenta racemosa, P. acris*].)

## BERGAMOT (*CITRUS BERGAMIA*)

This essence is expressed from the fruit rind of the bergamot tree. Its pleasant scent makes it popular as a fragrance and a highly compatible ingredient in many essential oil blends (e.g., with lavender or geranium). Bergamot is also a favorite flavoring in pastries, tea, confections, and medicines. Its genuinely deodorizing effects derive from its antiseptic properties, which are also effective against urinary infections. But its primary value is as a stomachic to treat gastric or digestive problems. Bergamot increases or restores proper appetite and, as a carminative, relieves flatulence. Its antispasmodic action also relieves colic, even as its antiparasitic properties make it an effective vermifuge. Bergamot also earns its reputation as a treatment for skin disorders, such as acne, when applied in a lotion or cream. Direct (neat) application of bergamot may, however, result in skin irritation or increase photosensitivity. The psychological effects of bergamot are as a sedative for anxiety and as an antidepressant. Its refreshing quality relieves melancholia. Bergamot can be used by means of baths, compresses, massage, or inhalation.

# CARDAMOM
# (*ELLETARIA CARDAMOMUM, AMOMUM AFZELII*)

Possessing an intense, sweet and spicy aroma, cardamom oil is steam distilled from the fruit (shells and seeds) of the *Elletaria cardamomum* indigenous to Asia or from the white almonds of *Amomum afzelii*. A botanical relative of ginger, cardamom has gained its own status and popularity as a flavoring agent and distinctive fragrance component. Other related species of cardamom (e.g., *Amomum cardamomum*, "Siam cardamom") are similarly used as spices or for therapeutic purposes, some as essential oils.

Stimulative, carminative, stomachic, and diuretic, cardamom is a superior appetite enhancer and digestive aid indicated for colic, dyspepsia, nausea, flatulence, gastric ulcers ("heartburn"), diarrhea, and similar maladies. It is particularly effective as a deodorant remedy for halitosis arising from gastric fermentation or from odoriferous foods such as garlic. Cardamom is antiseptic and also stimulates the phagocytic activity of the immune system. As a nerve tonic, cardamom is useful in the treatment of sciatica. Indeed, its positive nervine and cephalic properties have a brightening psychological influence.

# CARROT SEED (*DAUCUS CAROTA*)

The light yellow to amber colored essential oil distilled from the seeds (mostly in France, Egypt, and India) differs from the orange carrot oil produced from the root of the common edible carrot. Carrot seed oil nonetheless offers the same familiar scent. Diuretic and hepatic, carrot seed operates as a kidney and liver cleanser, particularly indicated for jaundice and hepatitis. Its depurative (detoxifying) properties are likewise effective for treating arthritis and rheumatism. As a diuretic remedy for genito-urinary ailments, carrot seed is indicated for gout, cystitis, and calculi as well as edema. Carrot seed stimulates lymphatic circulation and is otherwise carminative and vermifuge, and an emmenagogic menstrual regulator. Its relaxing qualities are helpful in the treatment of premenstrual tension. It is also considered a blood tonic indicated for anemia.

As a dermal agent, carrot seed lends its depurative qualities to skin and body care preparations and procedures. A natural tanning agent and skin toner that protects aged and wrinkled skin, carrot seed is also remedial for dermatitis, eczema, psoriasis, and various rashes. It can be used topically to treat boils, abscesses, and skin ulcers. Carrot seed oil is a fine ingredient for creams and lotions.

## CHAMOMILE, GERMAN
## (*MATRICARIA CHAMOMILLA*)

The essential oil is extracted from the flowers, which impart the sweet apple-like aroma so familiar to chamomile tea drinkers. German chamomile is a lovely blue color because of the greater quantity of azulene formed during distillation. Azulene (chamazulene) is a fatty substance possessing fine healing and anti-inflammatory properties effective in treating various conditions, from eczema, pruritus, and hives to gastritis, cystitis, and colitis. It is also strongly antibacterial, and so has been isolated for pharmaceutical use.

German chamomile's properties are quite like those of the Roman variety, except that its higher azulene content makes German chamomile more effectively bactericidal (e.g., as a superior wash for wounds and sores) and immunostimulant, whereby it strengthens leukocytes (white blood cells). It otherwise has similar antispasmodic, analgesic, antipyretic, sudorific, sedative, cholagogic, and vasoconstrictive capabilities and properties. Generally, what is said of the one chamomile is true for the other, but German chamomile is more highly prized as an ingredient in body and skin care preparations. It is also more often used as a topical remedy for severe skin afflictions or as an emmenagogue in the treatment of female reproductive disorders such as dysmenorrhea or amenorrhea. Its distinctive ability to reduce excessive blood urea makes it a preferable treatment for gout or nephritis. For that reason, too, it is a superior lymph and liver detoxifier.

## CHAMOMILE, ROMAN (*ANTHEMIS NOBILIS*)

The yellowish essential oil is produced by steam distillation of the plant's flowers and leaves, during which its important azulene constituent is formed. Because of its hydrating, anti-inflammatory, and antibacterial properties, chamomile is a widely used topical treatment for numerous skin disorders, such as burns, rashes, boils, acne, and dermatitis. It is used cosmetically to relieve skin pore congestion, principally by its solvent activity on sebum, and also as a hair lightener.

Chamomile is a remarkably versatile and effective remedy. Its antispasmodic, anticonvulsive, and antipyretic properties are helpful in treating cramps and fevers (ague). Stomachic and apéritif, chamomile is excellent for digestive sluggishness, colic, nausea, dyspepsia, and ulcers. As a hepatic stimulant (cholagogue), it is indicated in cases of jaundice and biliousness. Nervine and analgesic, chamomile provides relief for the pain and discomfort of gout, rheumatism, neuralgia, and toothache; also for migraine and earache, and any attendant symptoms of vertigo. Chamomile is likewise a soothing, anti-infectious remedy for gingivitis and an opthalmic treatment for conjunctivitis. It is known as a good blood tonic, helpful to the spleen and effectual in cases of anemia.

Chamomile's psychological influence as a mild sedative parallels its gentle and calming physiological effects, whether as a remedy for insomnia and anxiety or for hysteria and anger. It is suitable treatment for child tantrums and the hypersensitive behavior of menopause and premenstrual syndrome (PMS). Antidepressant, it relieves nightmares and moodiness as well as all choleric tempers. Of very low toxicity, chamomile is especially safe for childhood illnesses and is generally applied through massage, baths, compresses, masks, and inhalation.

# CLARY SAGE (*SALVIA SCLAREA*)

The essential oil steam distilled from the plant's herbs and flowers has traditionally been used in German muscatel wine, English beer, and Italian vermouth (as well as a perfume fixative) to exploit the heady effects and sensuous aroma of clary sage. Having deodorizing, anti-infectious, anti-inflammatory, and astringent yet sudorific properties, clary sage is also a valuable ingredient in body care preparations, whereby it regulates skin and hair secretions and acts as a scalp stimulant. It has opthalmic uses, too.

Clary sage is nervine with sedative effects. It lends its anticonvulsive, antispasmodic properties to the treatment of asthma. It lowers blood pressure, is a stomachic indicated for the treatment of dyspepsia and flatulence, and is a general tonic that blends well with juniper, lavender, or sandalwood for either stomach or kidney complaints. Clary sage relieves headache and vertigo and can be used to remedy sore throat or to treat menstrual difficulties requiring an emmenagogue. It works well in massage, baths, compresses, or inhalations.

Clary sage is an excellent relaxant having somewhat aphrodisiacal, euphoric, antidepressant characteristics especially helpful in the treatment of menopausal or PMS symptoms. A remedy for insomnia, it is likewise effectual for feelings of paranoia, panic, or hysteria. Specific conditions of neurasthenia or hyperactivity in children respond well to clary sage. Overuse can produce headache and may actually raise blood pressure, causing dizziness, rather than alleviate those conditions.

## CLOVE (*EUGENIA CARYOPHYLLATA*)

The pale yellow oil for aromatherapy is steam distilled from dried flower buds of the clove tree. It has a familiar hot, spicy aroma recognizable from clove's worldwide popularity as a preservative spice and food flavoring. Clove also appears in beverages and tobacco mixtures. Clove bud oil is a favorite top note in perfumery and a fragrance ingredient in various toiletries, cosmetics, toothpastes, and soaps. (*Note:* A less desirable yellow oil resembling clove bud is sometimes produced from clove stems. Even less suitable is the cruder brown oil from clove leaves.)

While principally known as an aperitive and stomachic condiment, clove has numerous other therapeutic virtues. First, its stimulative nature and wide-spectrum antimicrobial properties make clove an effective treatment for a multitude of digestive disorders, from dyspepsia to diarrhea. Clove is a carminative parasiticidal vermifuge that stimulates intestinal peristalsis, killing intestinal worms as it expels them. Topically applied, clove destroys the scabies mite and is an excellent fungicide for athlete's foot. Powerfully antiseptic, it can be used to disinfect wounds.

Antiviral and bactericidal, clove prevents contagion, which explains its extensive historical usage to combat plagues. For example, it has proved particularly effective against *Mycobacterium tuberculosis* and is also a treatment for measles, for which its antipyretic properties are likewise valuable. Clove is indicated for urinary infections as well as for gout and edema. It is good treatment for respiratory ills such as asthma, bronchitis, and pleurisy. Antispasmodic and antineuralgic, clove oil is a famous analgesic dentifrice for toothache, usually applied directly on a soaked cotton. It can be used to create a highly disinfectant mouthwash or gargle for throat and sinus ills that is also effective for halitosis arising either from tooth decay or stomach fermentation.

The chemical constituents of clove have been shown to be anticarcinogenic. In a 5 to 10 percent alcohol solution, clove is used to treat the skin lesions of lupus erythematosus (lupus vulgaris) and is similarly effective for measles rash and acne. The amazing versatility of clove extends to its many applications: inhalation, ingestion, massage, tincture, or other methods. Psychologically, clove is arousing and fortifying. A remedy for impotence or frigidity, it stimulates the libido by directly stimulating the reproductive genital organs. Clove is an equally energizing mental stimulant whose clarifying effects are especially helpful in cases showing symptoms of dizziness or vertigo. For all aromatherapy or other purposes, only clove bud oil should be used, and to minimize potential toxicity, moderate, low-dosage use is strongly emphasized. Irritation or sensitization of the skin or mucous membranes is possible from clove, and although it has a traditional reputation as an aid before and during childbirth, such use cannot be recommended without proper qualified supervision.

## CYPRESS (*CUPRESSUS SEMPERVIRENS*)

The clear to slightly yellow oil is distilled usually from the leaves of the tree and sometimes from the flowers, cones, nuts, and twigs. It has a woody, somewhat harsh aroma reminiscent of juniper. Cypress is primarily known for its antisudorific, astringent, and styptic properties capable of arresting excessive bodily secretions, ranging from diarrhea to bleeding. It has a vasoconstrictive activity similar to that of witch hazel (probably owing to its tannin content), which makes it a good remedy for hemorrhoids and vascular problems. Its antispasmodic properties provide additional benefits for menstrual and urinary difficulties involving pain and excessive flow, such as menorrhagia, enuresis, and incontinence. As an antibacterial, deodorizing skin treatment, cypress also helps dissolve and regulate oily sebaceous secretions. Cypress's vasoconstrictive properties suggest that its use by people who are hypertensive ought to be accompanied by some caution.

Cypress seems to have a special affinity for the female reproductive system. An estrogen stimulant, it has ovarian hormonal properties that recommend its use for gynecologic purposes. Cypress's antiseptic, antispasmodic features function well in sprays and gargles for the flu, laryngitis, and cough. Cypress blends well with pine, juniper, or sandalwood in baths, in compresses, or for inhalation from vaporizers and diffusors, whereby its soothing and relaxing characteristics can have their psychological effect as well. It is indicated for anxiety, confusion, or indecision coupled with impatience and irritability.

## EUCALYPTUS
## (*EUCALYPTUS CITRIODORA, E. GLOBULUS*)

Eucalyptus is one of the universal, i.e., most versatile, essential oils. It is steam distilled from the leaves of the eucalyptus tree, of which there are several hundred varieties. *Eucalyptus globulus* has a strong camphorous odor, largely owing to its 80 percent eucalyptol content. It is valuable as an inhalant, as a chest rub, and in massage, saunas, baths, and compresses for numerous ailments. An effective remedy for all respiratory ills, eucalyptus both deodorizes and inhibits contagion when used as a disinfectant. It relieves cough as both an expectorant and a decongestant, and it is an excellent treatment for sore throat and sinus problems. It can also treat urinary infections, although large doses can tax the kidneys. Antiseptic (bactericidal) and fungicidal, eucalyptus is moreover an effectual vermifuge. It is particularly indicated for its antidiabetic properties. *Eucalyptus globulus* is noted as an analgesic for migraine, rheumatism, and other muscle pain. It has a balancing yet reinvigorating psychological influence. *Eucalyptus citriodora* has a sedative effect. Known for its distinctive lemony scent, it is a first-rate sanitary disinfectant, deodorizer, or deodorant with both germicidal and antiparasitic powers. Like all eucalyptus, it is an insect repellent. It also has anti-inflammatory and toning properties that are excellent for the skin.

## EVERLASTING
## (*HELICHRYSUM ITALICUM, H. ANGUSTIFOLIUM*)

Also known as immortelle, everlasting is a recent newcomer to aromatherapy. There are several *Helichrysum* species. The essential oil can be distilled from the whole plant of this aromatic herb, which is widely cultivated in the Mediterranean, but is more ordinarily distilled from the fresh flowers or flowering tops. It is a popular fixative in fragrancing. An absolute/concréte of everlasting is used for tobacco flavoring.

Generally depurative, everlasting is a cholagogue specifically useful for relieving hepatic congestion and the resultant "liver headache" or migraine.

It strengthens the immune system and assists lymph drainage, which makes it a natural component for massage. Everlasting's anti-inflammatory (antiphlogistic) properties compare to those of its botanical cousin chamomile and are especially valuable to a variety of skin care procedures. Moreover, everlasting is cytophylactic (cell regenerative) with antiseptic, anti-allergenic, and astringent properties beneficial to the healing of wounds, burns, and bruises, as well as skin conditions such as acne, psoriasis, and eczema. Everlasting is a styptic (for external hemorrhaging) and a cicatrisant that reduces scarring. It makes a useful compress for sprains and neuralgia, and it is an expectorant for respiratory ailments, coughs, and congestions. An antidepressant, everlasting is likewise soothing for many stress-related psychological complaints. It relieves fatigue and as a nervine has a grounding influence upon nervous conditions. Everlasting reportedly increases dream activity.

## FENNEL (*FOENICULUM VULGARE*)

"Sweet fennel," a traditional culinary substance and food flavoring with a delicious aroma much like that of aniseed, offers a distilled essential oil from its own crushed seeds and from its roots and leaves as well. An ingredient of many liqueurs, fennel is also included in dentifrices and mouthwash to aid the gums. It is also found in cough drops and syrups.

Fennel's therapeutic properties are similar to those of its cousin aniseed, but fennel is generally considered to be medicinally safer. Stomachic and carminative, fennel has a normalizing effect as a digestive tonic for the liver and spleen and as a digestive aid for dyspepsia and nausea. Fennel tea is quite popular for digestive ills. Anthelmintic (vermifuge) and laxative, fennel is also an effective diuretic for oliguria (caused by either the suppression or retention of urine) and antilithic for dissolving renal calculi. An antispasmodic, it is an effective hiccough remedy and treatment for colic. As an apéritif, fennel's normalizing or regulating qualities operate to curb excessive appetite. This, combined with its capabilities as a diuretic and hormonal regulator, makes fennel effective for obesity.

Fennel is estrogenic, hence valuable in the treatment of menstrual irregularities and the psychosomatic conditions of PMS or menopausal syndrome. A galactagogue, fennel, like aniseed, promotes lactation. Fennel's hepatic detoxifying properties make it a useful hangover remedy and antidote to alcoholic poisoning from intoxication. In such cases, fennel has shown tissue regenerative powers. Its depurative and diuretic capabilities are mutually efficacious in cases of gout. The use of fennel to improve eyesight has a centuries-old history in both Europe and Asia. It is also said to reverse hearing loss. Its other opthalmic uses include the treatment of conjunctivitis and blepharitis.

When used as a hair rinse, fennel imparts luster and sheen. Another cosmetic use of fennel takes advantage of its depurative powers in cellulite treatments. Fennel is an excellent addition to massage, baths, or compresses. Psychologically, it lends confidence, strength, and courage. Although sweet fennel is relatively safe compared with aniseed (or, for that matter, bitter fennel) the wrong use of it may actually increase nervousness, apprehension, and anxiety. In those predisposed, such as epileptics, internal overdose could cause convulsions (the inverse effect of aniseed, which can be stupefacient). Children of preschool age are far more susceptible than adults to toxic effects from the internal use of fennel. Otherwise, sweet fennel is generally regarded as safe when administered moderately and correctly.

## FRANKINCENSE
## (*BOSWELLIA THURIFERA, B. CARTERI*)

Also known as olibanum, this legendary incense and "gift of the Magi" derives from the tree resin, a whitish gum, which is dissolved and distilled to obtain the essential oil. It is a premier and expensive ingredient in cosmetics and toiletries, typically as a fixative, because of its marvelous, exquisite scent and properties—most notably as a dry skin treatment that rejuvenates and tones while softening wrinkles and stretch marks. Antiseptic and astringent, frankincense is indicated for all male and female genitourinary infections and conditions. It is said to share many of the characteristics of myrrh and blends well with many other essences. In baths with juniper, for example, it is a good remedy for hemorrhoids or cystitis. As an expectorant inhalant for lung ailments and catarrhal conditions, frankincense is especially therapeutic for the mucous membranes. It has long been used in Ayurvedic medicine to treat a variety of inflammations, including arthritis and related rheumatic musculoskeletal diseases, as well as sores, ulcers, boils, and ringworm.

The psychologically relaxing, reassuring characteristics of frankincense are nicely disclosed in massage or steam inhalation, whereby tension and anxiety are gently alleviated. Frankincense has a grand and venerable reputation as an antidepressant for states of melancholia and morbidity—i.e., to vanquish "evil spirits." Its clinical ability to regulate and deepen respiration—a prerequisite for meditation and other spiritual exercises—further substantiates its traditionally important role in ceremonial and liturgical services.

## GERANIUM (*PELARGONIUM GRAVEOLENS*)

The essential oil is steam distilled from the entire plant, more often from the leaves. Geranium is another of aromatherapy's universal oils. Its aesthetic appeal as a fragrance is well known. Its many and marvelous therapeutic uses range from healing wounds to repelling insects. Geranium is an effective astringent, antiseptic, and diuretic. The oil is a good remedy for urinary ills and, like cinnamon and eucalyptus, is known for having antidiabetic properties. Its antimicrobial powers work well in a mouthwash or gargle for sore throat and other oral infections. Geranium is also valuable for all skin care treatments. It is active against yeasts, heals sores and burns, remedies dry skin and scalp, and helps smooth lines and wrinkles. Moreover, geranium relieves cramps and is a good aid for insect bites. It lends itself to virtually all therapeutic methods, including massage, baths, compresses, inhalation from vaporizers and diffusors, and various topical applications. For all purposes it blends well with lavender. Geranium is known to work on the cortex of the adrenal glands, which partly explains its ability to relieve nervousness, weariness, and depression. As a stimulant, its psychological effects are balancing and stabilizing, not sedative.

## GINGER (*ZINGIBER OFFICINALE*)

A native of Asia, ginger is one of the world's oldest and most renowned medicinal spices. Used in cooking and pastries, ginger is also the familiar constituent of ginger beer, ginger ales, and certain brandies and other beverages, as well as a popular fragrance ingredient. The essential oil is distilled from the roots of the ginger plant.

Laxative, tonic, stomachic, and apéritif, ginger is a fine remedy for loss of appetite, flatulence, and various indigestions. It reduces the nausea of motion sickness by its aromatic, carminative, and internally detoxifying effects. Analgesic, sudorific, and rubefacient, ginger applied in compresses, liniments, or by massage relieves backache, headache, and muscular or rheumatic pain. In Japan, ginger has traditionally been used to treat spinal and joint ailments and to promote healing of fractures. In China, ginger tea is a remedy for colds, coughs, flu, dysentery, and diarrhea. Ginger is a phagocyte immunostimulant. Antiseptic as well as febrifuge, it makes an effective sore throat gargle. It is hypertensive, and its fiery nature acts as an aphrodisiac for male impotence. Psychologically, too, ginger's stimulative and fortifying effects clear the mind even as it clears and promotes physical circulation. Owing to its strong rubefacient properties, ginger may be a skin irritant to some people.

## GRAPEFRUIT (*CITRUS PARADISI*)

Like other citrus oils, grapefruit is expressed from the fruit rind. Similarly, grapefruit shares with lemon and other citrus oils astringent and antiseptic properties, as well as stomachic and hepatic attributes that aid digestion. Indeed, grapefruit's distinguished reputation as a weight-loss agent originates from its solvent effect on fat and its diuretic relief of water retention. Grapefruit is both a gallstone solvent and a liver tonic; it is also a lymphatic stimulant and regulator. Its extract components and vitamin C content make grapefruit useful as an antimicrobial preservative. Grapefruit is a pleasant diffusor oil, having delightfully cool, refreshing, and uplifting antidepressant effects. When used topically it may sometimes cause photosensitivity.

## JASMINE
## (*JASMINUM OFFICINALE, J. GRANDIFLORUM*)

The celebrated "king of essences," jasmine is invariably one of the two or three most expensive oils and most precious of perfume components. Virtually every fragrance uses the exquisitely scented jasmine as a base note. The exorbitant price of jasmine oil—a pound of jasmine oil may cost as much as $3,000 to $4,000—is largely attributable to the complex, painstaking, and time-consuming process by which it is produced. It takes forty pounds of petals to create one ounce of essence—a minimum $75 value. It takes some 8 million jasmine flowers to produce each kilogram of oil. These blossoms must be gathered prior to sunrise so that the daylight will not adversely affect jasmine's bloom and extraordinarily fragrant essence, which peaks in the early hours before sunrise. Originally, the viscous jasmine absolute was extracted from the lovely white flowers by enfleurage. Today, it usually is more cheaply, and less suitably, extracted by solvents. A solvent extracted concréte is then transformed into jasmine absolute by alcohol separation. Sometimes an essential oil is further produced by distillation of the absolute. Fortunately, the concentrated strength of jasmine requires only tiny dosages, somewhat mitigating the high cost one must pay for the oil.

The therapeutic use of jasmine is primarily for physical complaints having a more immediate psychological origin. Jasmine is recognized as a good remedy for bronchial and respiratory ailments, such as catarrh, cough, and hoarseness, but its high cost is prohibitive for such common purposes, especially since there are other less expensive oils that are more effective— although jasmine tea, nearly as famous as the oil, is sometimes employed for such purposes. Like rose, jasmine has an affinity for the female reproductive system. It is a stabilizing tonic and nervine for menstrual discomfort and for the uterine pains of childbirth. Jasmine is a galactagogue as well as an antispasmodic. It is prized as a superior facial skin oil for both its anti-inflammatory and its cicatrisant properties. Generally too thick for diffusor use, jasmine can be inhaled or enjoyed in massage or baths.

Jasmine's benefits for psychosomatic ills derive from its antidepressant and euphoric characteristics. It is a psychotherapeutic remedy for forms of anxiety, panic, simple fear, or complex paranoia as well as hypochondria and apathy. Warmly reassuring, jasmine bolsters confidence and optimism. Its sensually romantic qualities are an ideal aphrodisiac for frigidity. Jasmine has a soulful nature that is profoundly inspirational.

## JUNIPER (*JUNIPERUS COMMUNIS*)

The colorless to pale greenish yellow oil is extracted by steam distillation from the berries (sometimes with the leaves and branches) of the familiar evergreen bush or small tree. Having a somewhat bitter taste and turpentine-like aroma, juniper is a popular additive to gin, both for flavoring and for its tonic effect upon the liver and digestion. Juniper is also diuretic and a kidney restorative, useful for kidney disturbances involving albuminuria and diabetes. In fact, like sandalwood, juniper is a first-rate remedy for most genito-urinary disorders. Generally, juniper makes an invaluable contribution to any efforts toward detoxification. It reduces uric acid in the blood, helping to reduce the aches and pains from gout, rheumatism, and arthritis. Juniper is effectual in all circulatory complaints, such as varicosity, hypertension, edema, et al. It is preventative for both kidney and bilious calculi. (When misused, juniper can overstimulate diseased or inflamed kidneys.) Juniper blends nicely with lavender and frankincense, or with cypress (its botanical cousin). In massage or bath, especially mixed with bergamot or cedarwood, juniper is a relief for cystitis.

Many skin problems, such as acne and eczema, respond to juniper in compresses or masks. Stomachic and carminative, it remedies colic. Antiseptic, juniper is useful as a household disinfectant or as a cough remedy or inhalant. Juniper's refreshingly stimulating, antidepressant nature dispels apathy, paranoia, confusion, or anxiety. Nervous states of paralysis or trembling also respond favorably to juniper.

## LAVENDER (*LAVANDULA OFFICINALIS*)

Lavender is a most remarkable universal oil, the many and varied uses for which seem almost too good to be true. It is by reputation the most versatile essential oil in aromatherapy. Steam distilled from flower heads, lavender oil is highly desirable as a fragrance and deodorant owing to its delicate and delightful scent. It is also renowned as a calming, soothing skin treatment for all kinds of skin problems and irritations. Lavender reduces puffiness and skin inflammation. Its value as a burn remedy is well documented. It prevents pore congestion and is effective against acne, especially in tandem with bergamot. The same anti-inflammatory properties that make lavender helpful for burns and abrasions are likewise useful for sunburn. Lavender is a cooling agent in cases of sunstroke or heat prostration. Cosmetically, it is a skin regenerator. It has insect repellent powers and is considered an anti-venom treatment for bites and stings. Lavender's analgesic qualities indicate its use for headaches, particularly for migraines, and the accompanying symptoms of dizziness and nausea. It works well as an antirheumatic ingredient in massage. All respiratory and sinus conditions respond to lavender, which is also an excellent aerosol disinfectant. It is a fungicide as well as an antiseptic or germicide and is therefore effective against an assortment of infectious problems, including vaginal disorders such as leukorrhea. Lavender lends itself to virtually all methods of usage and blends very well with other essential oils. Its antispasmodic abilities are medically applied to relieve heart palpitations and tachycardia. Lavender helps lower blood pressure. By its action upon the cerebrospinal nervous system it is a helpful treatment for neurasthenia and insomnia. The psychological effects of lavender are restorative and relaxing—almost euphoric. It is a fine anti-stress remedy for moods of impatience, irritability, and extreme panic or hysteria.

## LEMON (*CITRUS LIMONUM*)

The oil is obtained by pressing the fruit peel. Its cool and refreshing fragrance bespeaks its antipyretic qualities. Lemon is known as a blood tonic and diuretic specifically good for circulatory ailments. It is also used for various ills of the liver and kidneys: to relieve congestions, prevent gallstones, and treat kidney stone conditions. Lemon is a stomachic that will regulate stomach acidity. Like all citrus, it has an alkaline effect in the system. It is good for dyspepsia. Lemon is an astringent skin toner that has a mild bleaching action and helps to reduce puffiness and wrinkles. It is an excellent massage remedy for lymphatic stasis or congestion and a cosmetic treatment to strengthen fingernails. Lemon is an effective aid for insect bites and stings and is antiparasitical, both internally and topically. Its antiseptic, bactericidal capacities recommend it as a respiratory remedy as well as a gargle or mouthwash for throat and gums. When it is inhaled, lemon's psychological effects are typically uplifting and reviving.

## LEMONGRASS
## (*ANDROPOGON* OR *CYMBOPOGON CITRATUS*)

The distilled essential oil obtained from this perennial tropical grass has a distinctive lemony fragrance less intense than that of citronella. There are several varieties of lemongrass, including chemotypes, producing a high yield to meet the high demand for this oil. Lemongrass is used in beverages and soaps, and it provides a top note in perfumery. Frequently, lemongrass is employed as an adulterant to stretch the more costly oils of melissa and lemon verbena.

Carminative and stomachic, lemongrass is a gastric stimulant useful for gastroenteritis and colitis. It has nervine properties that help regulate the autonomic (parasympathetic) nervous system. Analgesic, lemongrass is a headache remedy. It is also an excellent massage treatment; its further capacity to reduce lactic acid as well as to tone connective and vascular tissue greatly relieves aches and pains. Indeed, lemongrass is indicated for conditions of varicosity, whereby its astringent qualities help to reduce swelling. Lemongrass is also diuretic and has galactagogic properties as well. Its antipyretic characteristics make it an especially toning and refreshing febrifuge. The topical astringency and antiseptic features of lemongrass make it an effective cleanser for oily skin with acne, especially when combined with lavender as a buffering agent. Cautious use of lemongrass for skin care is necessary, however, because topical overdose or neat application may cause dermal irritation. Lemongrass should be adequately diluted or used sparingly; two or three drops will suffice.

Lemongrass is antimicrobial and a phagocyte immunostimulant; it resists contagion when employed as an aerosol disinfectant or other means of vaporization. It is a good sanitary disinfectant as well. Like its botanical cousin, citronella, lemongrass is a first-rate insect repellent and parasiticide. The bactericidal properties of lemongrass have been shown to be more effective against *Staphylococcus aureus* than those of either penicillin or streptomycin. Lemongrass is a treatment for athlete's foot and can be used in a foot bath for sore, sweaty, and especially odoriferous feet. For either general or localized offensive body odor (bromidrosis), lemongrass makes an especially refreshing deodorant bath treatment. For such purposes, of course, the same cautions about dermal and mucous membrane sensitization or irritation apply. Psychologically, lemongrass is equally refreshing; its antidepressant qualities assist mental clarity and acuity.

## MANDARIN (*CITRUS RETICULATA*)

The oil is expressed from the fruit peel. Mandarin is not regarded as a major essential oil, but it does blend and work well with other citrus oils and is especially valuable in massage. Its delicate and popular fragrance adds to its gentle tonic and stimulant effects. Mandarin is a primary remedy for stomach and liver problems. Its sedative and antispasmodic capabilities make it a quite suitable remedy for hiccough, belching, and heart palpitations associated with gas pressure or thoracic and stomach spasms. Mandarin is similarly useful for bouts of nausea, cramps, morning sickness, and constipation. It reduces high blood pressure and offers effective relief for depression and melancholia.

# MARJORAM (*ORIGANUM MARJORANA, MARJORANA HORTENSIS*)

The essential oil is distilled from all parts of the plant, especially the flowering heads. Marjoram has earned esteem as a healing herb and digestive aid. Its fine flavor and antimicrobial (antibacterial, fungicidal) properties have made marjoram a traditionally popular food spice. It is carminative and laxative, therefore valuable in weight control by reducing bloating, flatulence, and constipation and by increasing peristalsis. Generally, marjoram relieves intestinal and menstrual cramps and swelling. It is hypotensive and vasodilating, helping to disperse bruises. It is an antispasmodic expectorant, useful in cases of bronchitis and for head congestion and catarrh or sinusitis. Marjoram is a good analgesic for rheumatoid pain, migraine, and body sprains.

A special use for marjoram is as an anaphrodisiac for compulsive, excessive sexual behavior. Marjoram is also known as a heating, fortifying antidepressant. A tranquilizing sedative, it has value as a treatment for anxiety, nervous irritability, grief, and associated insomnia. Marjoram has a variety of applications, including baths, compresses, massage, infusions, and inhalation, but some caution is necessary because it may induce drowsiness if wrongly used. Marjoram should be avoided during early pregnancy.

# MYRRH (*COMMIPHORA* OR *BALSAMODENDRON MYRRHA*)

One of the Magi's three gifts to the infant Jesus, myrrh's mystical reputation is nearly equal to that of its cousin, frankincense. The essential oil is distilled from the gum or oleoresin of the myrrh bush (or small tree) found throughout the Middle East and northeast Africa. Owing to its exceptional preservative (antiseptic, antiputrescent) properties, myrrh was used in Egypt for embalming. Despite its harsh, pungent odor, and equally bitter taste, myrrh's natural viscosity and unique qualities make it a favorite fixative (base) in perfumery. Furthermore, it blends very well with frankincense, sandalwood, or patchouli, as with many other oils.

Antiseptic, antiphlogistic, and astringent, myrrh is a first-rate wound and ulcer healer. As a tincture or wash it can be used effectively for all mouth and throat afflictions, benefiting the teeth and gums and combating thrush, gingivitis, pyorrhea, and laryngitis. Expectorant and anticatarrhal, myrrh has many pulmonary applications, including treatment of bronchitis and chest colds. It prevents or inhibits contagion. Fungicidal, it makes a good vaginal douche for leukorrhea and a good remedy for athlete's foot. Applied topically, myrrh is a treatment for ringworm and an excellent drying agent for eczema and psoriasis. It is a prized ingredient in facial applications for stretch marks and wrinkles, and generally its balsamic, cooling, and toning properties are corrective for piles and diarrhea. Stomachic and carminative, myrrh helps combat gastrointestinal fermentations.

Myrrh is a good constituent of massage therapy, and although its viscosity prevents ready dissolution in baths or diffusors, it is an excellent inhalant. Its primary psychological characteristic is sedative, but myrrh also fortifies the etheric energy or body aura and helps deepen meditation, which explains why it is traditionally included in incense for liturgical services. Traditionally, myrrh has proven useful as an emmenagogue for menstrual difficulties such as amenorrhea, and as a uterine tonic and regulator in obstetrics, but its unqualified use during pregnancy cannot be endorsed.

## NEROLI (*CITRUS VULGARIS, C. BIGARADIA*)

Also known as orange blossom (*Citrus aurantium* var. *amara*), neroli oil can be produced by enfleurage, solvent extraction, or most desirably by steam distillation from the fresh flowers of the bitter (or sour) orange tree found in the Mediterranean. Neroli exemplifies the wonderful versatility of orange trees. An inferior but useful essential oil is likewise produced from the sweet orange (*Citrus aur.* var. *dulcis* or *Citrus sinensis*) and orange oils can be cold pressed from the skin of either variety. Also, petitgrain is obtained from the tips (branches and leaves) of the *Citrus aur.* var. *amara*. Neroli is an expensive oil, prized as a fixative in perfumery because of its exquisitely sweet scent. (It takes approximately a ton of orange blossoms to produce one quart of neroli oil.) It also offers an excellent orange floral water (aromatic hydrosol). Unsurprisingly, neroli is often stretched (adulterated) with less expensive oils.

A digestive aid and soothing intestinal carminative, neroli is a valuable remedy for cases of diarrhea, cramps, colic, and nervous stomach. Antispasmodic and hypotensive, neroli restores natural cardiac rhythm and so is indicated for tachycardia, palpitations, and assorted cardiac contractions or spasms. For example, it alleviates false angina linked to anxiety. Antiseptic and cell rejuvenating, neroli is a valuable skin care for all skin types, especially sensitive, inflamed, or dry skin. It is an effective vascular treatment for spider veins and is cicatrisant for scars. Neroli is a useful germicidal deodorant, and its unique properties add much to a relaxing bath. Massage and inhalation are other methods whereby neroli's psycho-physiological benefits can be derived.

Neroli is antidepressant, sedative, and soporific, hence suitable to a wide variety of psychological afflictions, ranging from insomnia and melancholia to anxiety and nervousness, from simple stage fright or performance jitters to hypersensitivity, PMS, desperation, and emotional shock or trauma. Neroli is renowned as a somewhat hypnotic aphrodisiac that relieves first-encounter apprehensions. That is why orange blossom has been the traditional flower of bridal bouquets for generations. Neroli is noteworthy for its safety in all applications.

## NIAOULI (*MELALEUCA VIRIDIFLORA*)

This botanical cousin of cajeput, eucalyptus, and tea tree offers a pale to dark yellow oil distilled from its twigs and leaves. Niaouli is also known as gomenol. It is a vermifuge and generally anti-infectious, therefore effectual for a variety of urinary and intestinal diseases. Niaouli is a non-irritating antiseptic, which, unlike cajeput, is gentle to the skin and mucous membranes. Like cypress, it soothes oily skin. An expectorant, niaouli is an excellent remedy for catarrhal respiratory or bronchial ailments, as well as for sinus problems and as a mouthwash or throat gargle. It is useful in obstetrics and gynecology; for example, as a douche. Niaouli has tissue regenerative properties that specifically increase tissue oxygenation and thereby counter the effects of smoking and air pollution and greatly aid the healing of wounds, burns, and ulcers. Especially when used in massage or inhaled, niaouli's psychological effects may range from balancing to stimulating. Overuse may actually increase agitation.

## PALMAROSA (*CYMBOPOGON MARTINI*)

This aromatic grass from the same family as lemongrass and citronella yields a yellow oil having a cross-scent reminiscent of rose and geranium. Palmarosa is primarily used in cosmetology and perfumery, often to stretch (i.e., adulterate) genuine rose oil. It is an antiseptic skin regenerator and hydrating (moisturizing) skin treatment for dry or aged skin, wrinkles, and general skin disturbances. Palmarosa regulates sebum production and is a remedy for minor skin infections. Otherwise its medicinal value is as a digestive aid and tonic.

## PATCHOULI (*POGOSTEMON CABLIN*)

Steam distilled from the leaves of the plant, patchouli oil carries a strong, distinctive fragrance that people either despise or adore. It is an extremely popular perfume in India, from whence it has gained its fame and exotic reputation as an aphrodisiac. Less is known about its therapeutic properties. It has value as a diuretic and anti-inflammatory agent as well as a remedy for certain poisonous bites and stings. It is fungicidal and cytophylactic (cell regenerative), useful for wound healing, skin care, and skin conditions such as dermatitis, eczema, athlete's foot, seborrhea, and dandruff. Patchouli has an arousing quality that provides an antidote for moods of apathy or indifference; it is likewise helpful for mental confusion or indecision. The benefits of patchouli are best derived through inhalation or topical application, especially from massage.

## PEPPER, BLACK (*PIPER NIGRUM*)

The pungent essential oil of this most used and famous food spice is obtained from peppercorns—the dried berries or seeds of the plant. Black pepper is antiviral, antispasmodic, rubefacient, and antipyretic. Also carminative and stomachic, it is a powerful digestive stimulant and effective remedy for dyspepsia, flatulence, nausea, and loss of appetite. Additionally, it provides antitoxin protection against food poisoning, such as from fish or mushrooms. It is likewise effective in cases of diarrhea and dysentery. A tonic for the spleen, black pepper is a blood stimulant, increasing both blood flow and production, and therefore indicated for certain kinds of anemia. It is a hypertensive useful for treating angina. Its antiseptic and analgesic properties make black pepper an excellent aid for head colds, sore throat, and toothache. When applied during massage, it also strengthens muscle tone. Black pepper's psychological influence is reassuring and fortifying. If overused for its diuretic capabilities, black pepper could irritate the kidneys.

# PEPPERMINT (*MENTHA PIPERITA*)

Steam distilled from the leaves and flower tops, peppermint oil has a sharp, refreshing scent recognizable by its menthol content. Peppermint is a particularly fast-acting general tonic, traditionally used as a digestive aid and remedy for dyspepsia, nausea, colic, and flatulence as well as a mouthwash and breath freshener. It has antispasmodic and analgesic properties that are most useful to relieve menstrual discomfort, toothache, headache, and sinus pain. Peppermint clears the head and one's thinking processes; its revivifying qualities are of great benefit for episodes of dizziness or fainting. The psychological effects of peppermint lift one's spirits out of a state of ennui or fatigue. Peppermint is good for the heart. Overuse can, however, lead to insomnia, or cause gastric irritation if overdone as a stomachic or carminative. When applied topically, peppermint's hot-cool sensation upon the skin can be disquieting to some, but it is generally useful for fever or hot flashes. Peppermint is indicated as a remedy for itching, but sometimes when used topically it can be the cause of the same. Its analgesic properties work nicely into massage treatments for muscle pain and neuralgia. External use for localized head or stomach pain is also effective. Peppermint is an antiseptic and decongestant suitable for all respiratory complaints. It mixes well with other oils as a treatment for colds and flu, also lending its sudorific properties and its ability to counter malaise. Peppermint is antiparasitic and an insect repellent. Known as a strongly effective inhalant, peppermint can be a pleasurable additional ingredient for saunas or steam baths.

# PETITGRAIN (*CITRUS VULGARIS, C. BIGARADIA*)

Also known as orange tree leaf, petitgrain essential oil is distilled from leaves (tips and twigs) of the same *Citrus aurantium* var. *amara* that produces neroli. Commonly used as a confection or pharmaceutical flavoring, petitgrain is also popular in the fragrance industry as a top note. Its refreshing flowery scent is lighter and more neutral than that of neroli. Petitgrain blends well with numerous other oils and is considered a less expensive, multipurpose alternative to neroli. Correspondingly, petitgrain bears a therapeutic resemblance to neroli, but its properties and effects—for example as a sedative or nervine—are usually less dramatic and less powerful. Petitgrain is similarly antiseptic and deodorant. As a stomachic, tonic digestive aid for dyspepsia or other gastric complaints, petitgrain is actually more stimulating than neroli. Cleansing, astringent, and antiperspirant, petitgrain is an excellent skin care treatment for greasy, weeping dermal conditions such as acne, eczema, and dermatitis. It makes a fine bath oil or shampoo rinse as well.

Psychologically, petitgrain is invigorating, uplifting, and clarifying. It is a heartening remedy for less profound or intense cases of stress-related anxiety, temporary disappointment, or sadness. Petitgrain is conspicuously safe to use and is especially effective in massage. (*Note:* There are other petitgrain oils produced from the tree leaves and twigs of lemon, bergamot, sweet orange, mandarin, and tangerine.)

## PINE (*PINUS SYLVESTRIS*)

Also known as Scots pine, this botanical cousin of juniper and cypress offers a clear to pale yellow essential oil with a familiar scent, most often distilled from the needles but also from the buds, resin of the tree (turpentine), pine cones, and twigs. Pine is considered a foremost remedy for all respiratory ills. It is an excellent inhalant (especially mixed with lavender and/or eucalyptus) for colds, catarrh, and sinusitis. Avicenna recommended it for pneumonia and lung infections. Expectorant and antiseptic, pine counters the effects of heavy smoking while increasing the oxygenation of tissues. It is highly effectual as a deodorizing disinfectant and works equally well as a genito-urinary antiseptic. Pine is a popular ingredient in many detergents, soaps, and bath preparations.

Pine is sometimes included in massage to increase circulation and relieve rheumatic pain. More often it is employed in steam inhalation, vaporizers, and diffusors, in which it blends nicely with tea tree and eucalyptus. Pine's psychological effects are bracing, strengthening, and stabilizing—an invigorating mental and adrenal stimulant. Also rubefacient, it has some tendency to irritate the skin.

## ROSE
## (*ROSA DAMASCENA, R. CENTIFOLIA, R. GALLICA*)

The three varieties of true rose yield two kinds of rose oil: (1) rose absolute, the standard rose essence, and (2) rose otto, or rose attar, the steam distilled essential oil. The otto (attar) is the more costly and rare of the two but also more useful to aromatherapy. Rose oil is perhaps the most famous and expensive perfume, which is why it is frequently stretched (adulterated) with other like-scented oils, most notably geranium and palmarosa. Traditionally regarded as the perfect flower, rose shares with jasmine the highest status in aromatherapy.

Virtually nontoxic, rose is antiseptic, anti-inflammatory, and astringent. It is a highly valued beauty oil in skin care. A cell regenerator and moisturizing cleanser for all skin types, rose is an excellent treatment for dry or inflamed skin conditions as well as for allergies and eczema. A remedy for vaginitis, it is also a female hormonal restorative and emmenagogue, useful for all uterine and menstrual infirmities. Rose is also indicated for sterility, impotence, and frigidity.

As a consummate purifying agent, rose's remarkable healing powers— extending to the cardiovascular, digestive, and nervous systems—are physiologically analogous to its symbolic reputation for completion and perfection. It is stomachic and laxative, choleretic and cholagogue—a superior cleansing tonic for the liver, countering the effects of alcohol and the symptoms of hangover. Rose has a positive influence on the heart rhythm and blood circulation. Its opthalmic use is for conjunctivitis and blepharitis. Rose is noted as the aphrodisiac of pure love and as a spiritually uplifting, gently euphoric antidepressant for all human passions of the heart, especially grief, jealousy, envy, sorrow, and disappointment.

## ROSEMARY (*ROSMARINUS OFFICINALIS*)

Rosemary oil is usually distilled from the flowering tops of the medicinal herb (sometimes the leaves or the whole plant). Its deserved reputation as a universal oil ought to be attended by a few cautions. Rosemary is potent, and its multitude of uses require some discrimination. It raises arterial pressure by liberating adrenaline from the adrenal cortex. Furthermore, the heavy use of rosemary could result in nervousness, spasms, or possibly convulsive reactions in those predisposed to such conditions, because of rosemary's dual effect upon the nerves and the adrenals. The hazards that rosemary might pose are attributable to overdose and overuse—temptations that sometimes arise because rosemary is such an extraordinary oil with superior characteristics and having so many marvelous uses that one is easily inclined to use it all the time. Indeed, rosemary is effective as an inhalant and in massage, compresses, baths, shampoos, and facials. It is a nervine, a diuretic, an analgesic, a rubefacient, and an astringent. It is an excellent treatment for all skin conditions, including wrinkles, acne, dermatitis, eczema, and dandruff. Rosemary's gifts as a skin and hair rejuvenator are greatly appreciated by dermatologists, cosmetologists, and aestheticians. Two rosemary chemotypes, *verbenon* and *cineol*, are notable for their abilities to improve the metabolism of the dermal layers. Therapeutically, rosemary is a heart tonic and a genuine boon to the liver and gallbladder, wherein it helps to regulate bile production. By its action it prevents bloating and constipation while normalizing the digestive and eliminative processes. Rosemary fights infection and relieves cramps, aches and pains, headaches, and flatulence. It heals burns and has both antitoxin and antiparasitical properties. Generally, it is considered to be an all-purpose remedy for respiratory and digestive ills. Psychologically, rosemary is energizing and uplifting. It reduces mental fatigue and strain while improving memory and thinking.

## ROSEWOOD (*ANIBA ROSAEODORA*)

Steam distilled from the wood chips of the tree, rosewood oil is not widely used for therapeutic purposes, and little research into its medicinal value has been done. Consequently, rosewood is too often neglected in aromatherapy. It has a positively wonderful scent that makes it popular as a fragrance and deodorant, and it is a favorite ingredient in many body and skin care products because of its cell-regenerative properties. Aside from limited antibacterial uses and as an occasional remedy for headache and nausea, rosewood's further advantages are psychological. It has a gentle and calming influence that nicely complements either a bath or a massage; it effectively clears the mind and evokes a feeling of well-being; and it has achieved distinction as a particularly sensuous aphrodisiac.

## SANDALWOOD (*SANTALUM ALBUM*)

The oil is obtained by steam distilling the heart wood. Sandalwood has a marvelous, slowly unfolding scent that has made it highly valued in the Orient as both a fragrance and an incense ingredient. Sandalwood is a mainstay of Indian yoga and meditation practices and of Ayurvedic medicine, in which it is employed for its diuretic and antiseptic properties in cases of urinary infection and venereal disease. Sandalwood is also a pulmonary antiseptic, useful for bronchitis. It has been successfully used as a skin treatment and topical astringent for conditions ranging from sensitive, inflamed skin to varicose veins and piles. Sandalwood is a popular ingredient in cosmetics, not only for its skin care benefits but also for its remarkable scent, which men and women both find pleasing. It is enjoyably effective as an inhalant by any aromatherapy method. Another of sandalwood's medical uses has been as a topical remedy for laryngitis and other throat afflictions; usually applied in compresses, it is not to be gargled. Sandalwood is an antidepressant and hormone regulator that, like rosewood, has gained fame as an aphrodisiac. In such capacities it has served as a remedy for both insomnia and impotence. Sandalwood has a euphoric yet grounding psychological effect that promotes a sense of well-being.

## SPIKENARD (*ARALIA RACEMOSA*)

The oil is obtained from the root by steam distillation. A traditional herbal ingredient of cough syrups, spikenard is known to be a stimulant tonic, diuretic, and cleansing blood purifier. It is an effective treatment for pulmonary diseases and also for gynecologic and venereal diseases. It has been used for leukorrhea and hemorrhoids and as a tea to lessen the pain of parturition. In massage or compresses it is a likewise effective aid for rheumatic pain and can also be used topically for skin eruptions. It relieves physical and emotional exhaustion. Spikenard should not be confused with the spike lavender (*Lavandula spica*) or aspic, which is a distinctly camphorous oil having its own valuable uses and properties. Spike lavender is an analgesic and cerebrospinal tranquilizer with antiseptic and rubefacient qualities. It is helpful in the treatment of burns and abscesses as well as an effective insecticide and bug repellent. Spike lavender is a good selection for sports massage, but it is not spikenard. (Neither is lavandin, an essential oil producing hybrid of true lavender and spike lavender.) There is an essential oil of sumbul or muskroot (*Nardostachius jatamansii*) that is referred to as spikenard. Sumbul oil is an especially exotic stabilizing fixative used in essential oil combinations and perfume mixtures. Its fragrant effects are grounding, but little or no research has been done regarding its therapeutic value.

# SPRUCE, BLACK (*PICEA MARIANA, P. NEGRA*)

The black spruce tree is a member of the vast and majestic Pinaceae plant family, which includes hemlock, fir, and pine. It yields a delightfully scented colorless oil distilled from its branches (needles and twigs). Black spruce's therapeutic properties and indications are similar to fir's, as is its fragrance, which is otherwise darker and more profound. Essential oils are, in fact, distilled from the twigs or needles of various *Pinaceae* trees—viz., *Abies* (fir), *Picea* (spruce), *Pinus* (pine), and *Tsuga* (hemlock)—which are generically, albeit imprecisely, referred to as "fir needle oil." Once again, the specific botanical names are instructive: e.g., Siberian fir (*Abies siberica*), Canadian fir (*Abies balsamea*), and white fir (*Abies alba*); or as examples of spruce: Norway spruce (*Picea abies*), white or Canadian spruce (*Picea glauca, P. alba, P. canadensis*). Like its relatives, black spruce is widely employed as a fragrance component and medicinal ingredient.

Antiseptic, expectorant, and antitussive, black spruce is an ideal remedy for all lung ailments (e.g., asthma and bronchitis) whether utilized as an inhalant or a cough remedy. Indeed, the vital etheric energy (prana) condensed and transmitted in and by black spruce effectively vibrates throughout the respiratory, nervous, and glandular systems of the human body. Black spruce is also a highly suitable remedy for genito-urinary complaints. Analgesic and rubefacient, black spruce is a powerful massage treatment for muscular or rheumatic aches and pains. It greatly stimulates circulation. It can be used in liniments, in diffusors, or as an aerosol disinfectant. Black spruce has a wonderfully penetrating fragrance that is said to enhance yoga or other meditations. Black spruce is a bracing, revitalizing tonic and steadying nervine. It is simultaneously elevating and grounding. Psychologically, it imparts fortitude and firm self-reliance.

# TEA TREE (*MELALEUCA ALTERNIFOLIA*)

Tea tree, or ti-tree, oil is a welcome newcomer to aromatherapy. It is acquired by steam distilling the leaves of the tree, and it has a medicinal odor somewhat reminiscent of its Australian cousin, the eucalyptus. Tea tree's most prominent feature is its extraordinary effectiveness against all three main infectious groups: fungi, bacteria, and viruses. It is a dynamic treatment for cold sores and other herpes; sinus and throat infections; respiratory ills; athlete's foot, ringworm, thrush, *Candida albicans*, and other yeast or fungal infections; genito-urinary disorders; such as *Trichomonas vaginalis* infection; and virtually every other infection or infestation included in the three groups. Tea tree's germicidal, antiparasitic, antifungal, and otherwise antimicrobial properties make it an extensively powerful wide-spectrum household disinfectant. Despite being virtually "anti–anything infectious," tea tree oil is also virtually nontoxic and hypoallergenic. It can be used freely in baths, steams, gargles, and mouthwashes. It can be inhaled through vaporization or diffusion, and it is beneficial in both massage and cosmetics. Tea tree is an effective remedy for skin and scalp disorders that involve infection or infestation or that require healing.

## VETIVER (*ANDROPOGON MURICATUS*)

A cousin to palmarosa, lemongrass, and citronella, vetiver yields a thick essential oil distilled from the roots of the grass. More often used as a fixative in perfumery than in aromatherapy, vetiver has a heavy, musky, earthy scent with lemony overtones.

Vetiver is a rubefacient of value in treating arthritis. A hormonal balancer with an affinity for female psychological problems connected with menopause, anorexia, and postpartum depression, vetiver is also a good remedy for nervousness and exhaustion. It is prized in skin care for its deep penetration, plumping up thin and sagging skin tissues. Vetiver has traditionally been used to repel moths. Its therapeutic properties operate well in massage, baths, lotions, and fragrances. Having a stimulating, yet grounding quality, vetiver provides a steadying, deepening effect.

## YARROW (*ACHILLEA MILLEFOLIUM*)

An extensive species of flowering herb widely found in global temperate zones, yarrow yields an azulene-rich, characteristically blue-green oil by steam distillation. Yarrow is sometimes used to stretch German chamomile.

Antiallergenic, anti-inflammatory, and astringent, yarrow is especially indicated as a skin and vascular tonic for many conditions of varicosity (e.g., hemorrhoids). A hypotensive blood cleanser, yarrow has beneficial effects upon various circulatory conditions, such as arteriosclerosis, high blood pressure, and thrombosis. Sudorific, antipyretic, and antispasmodic, yarrow is also a healing antiseptic treatment for various wounds, sores, ulcers, and lacerations. Moreover, it has styptic or hemostatic properties. Yarrow is equally effective for acne, rashes, and scars. It can be used to treat gynecological problems such as infection, pain, and irregular menses. As a shampoo rinse, it promotes hair growth. Yarrow nicely lends its therapeutic qualities to the methods of massage, inhalation, and compresses. Psychologically, yarrow eases tension and imparts a balancing influence during times of cyclical psychosomatic crisis or transition, such as puberty, menopause, and menstruation.

## YLANG YLANG (*CANANGA ODORATA*)

Obtained by steam distillation of the flowers from the tree, ylang ylang oil has a sweet, somewhat heady floral scent that reminds some people of mixed almond and jasmine. Ylang ylang is hypotensive and has the ability to help regulate cardiopulmonary rhythms; this makes it valuable as a treatment for high blood pressure, tachycardia, palpitations, and hyperventilation. Ylang ylang is found in skin care preparations, owing to its moisturizing effects, and in perfume mixtures. It is an aid for oily skin and a good scalp stimulant. Naturally, it also has some anti-infectious properties. But ylang ylang's highest distinction is as a psychological agent having antidepressant, sedative, and aphrodisiacal powers. Indeed, ylang ylang is known to be a fine treatment for frigidity and impotence. Its soporific and sedative capabilities make it an effectual counteragent for anxiety, angry or hysterical states, and insomnia. Heavy usage of ylang ylang could, however, cause headaches.

# Appendix

## FLORAL WATERS IN AROMATHERAPY

Floral waters are aromatherapy's best kept secret. Whereas pure essential oils are rightfully emphasized in the practice of aromatherapy, there are many therapeutic and aesthetic purposes for which floral waters (aromatic hydrosols) are actually more suitable and convenient.

A true floral water contains the plant's valuable water-soluble components that are infused into the distilled water during the steam distillation process customarily employed to extract the plant's essential oil. Therefore, aromatic hydrosols are milder than the concentrated oils. Accordingly, they are also less expensive. Floral waters are a more affordable way to gain many of the benefits otherwise derived from particularly costly precious oils such as chamomile, rose, and neroli.

Aromatic hydrosols are good for numerous topical applications, such as compresses and facials. Since they are the pure water distillates of fresh flowers and do not contain alcohol or any other additives, hydrosols are ideal skin toners, fresheners, and astringents.

## AROMATIC DIFFUSORS

A diffusor is a special air-pump device uniquely designed to dispense essential oils into the atmosphere. It is the most effective way to finely vaporize essential oils without harming or altering their vital components and valuable properties. Although there are other inhalation methods and techniques (e.g., steams, heat lamps, or the direct inhalation of a few drops of essential oil placed on a paper tissue), a diffusor is the easiest, most convenient way to experience the many benefits of essential oils and aromatherapy.

The primary components of a diffusor are the glass nebulizer and an air pump connected by flexible tubing, usually plastic. Designs vary, but the effects are generally alike. Only true essential oils should be used in a diffusor. Some essential oils are nonetheless unsuitable for diffusor use because of their thicker viscosity and lesser volatility. Others, such as sandalwood, vetiver, and patchouli, although more viscous, can be diluted in blends with less viscous oils to increase vaporization and avoid clogging the glass nebulizer. Nebulizers ought to be detached from the air pump before being cleaned periodically with alcohol.

As with any aromatherapy treatment method, one must exercise caution when using a diffusor near children, infants, or pets. Otherwise, the duration and frequency of diffusor use is a matter of personal preference, guided by one's experience and knowledge of essential oils.

## BASIC PRINCIPLES OF ESSENTIAL OIL BLENDING

Because they act synergetically, essential oils generally blend well. Successful blending of essential oils is, however, an acquired skill, requiring experience and knowledge of oils that complement one another both therapeutically and aesthetically. First is the matter of compatibility: mixing oils having contrary effects (e.g., calming versus stimulating) should be avoided. Your intention for the blend is of primary importance to your selection of oils, as is the intended method of usage. And, of course, you must always consider the person for whom you are selecting and blending the oils. From there, learn to follow your nose. Mixtures including 2 to 5 essential oils are recommended; mixing more than 5 or 6 oils in combination seldom adds to their cumulative effect and may actually detract from it.

# Charts and Tables

## AROMATHERAPY USAGE GUIDE

Follow these simple guidelines to create your own aromatherapy products. EO = singular essential oil or essential oil combination.

| USES | BLENDING AND APPLICATIONS |
| --- | --- |
| Baths | Mix 8 to 10 drops of pure EO into warm bath water, soak for 20 minutes, and rest for 1/2 hour. |
| Full Body Massage or Body Oil | Add 10 to 20 drops of pure EO per 1 ounce of a carrier oil, such as sweet almond, jojoba, canola, grapeseed, or apricot. |
| Partial Body Application | Add 20 to 40 drops of pure EO per 1 ounce carrier oil. |
| Inhalation | Place 2 to 5 drops of pure EO on a clean tissue, then inhale. |
| Diffusors | Use only pure EO. To avoid clogging your diffusor, particularly viscous EO should be either avoided or well diluted with lighter EO. |
| Facial Oil | Add 3 to 5 drops of pure EO to 1/2 ounce of facial oil or facial gel base. |

*Dry/devitalized skin types:* hazelnut oil; facial gel with liposomes; avocado oil with a small amount of borage and/or natural vitamin E.

*Imbalanced skin types:* apricot and/or jojoba oil with a small amount of rosehips seed oil.

As a relaxing evening treatment, thoroughly cleanse your face and gently massage a few drops of facial oil into your skin.

| | |
|---|---|
| Clay Facial Mask | First, mix 2 tablespoons of powdered clay into a selected liquid, such as distilled water, aromatic hydrosol, or fresh cucumber juice; then add 2 to 5 drops pure EO.<br><br>Apply clay mixture to clean skin, allow to dry, and rinse off thoroughly with tepid to cool water (do not use soap). Complete the treatment with an application of facial oil or nourishing facial gel. (Note: Always avoid eye areas when applying clay masks.) |
| Clay Partial Body Pack | First, mix 1/4 to 1/2 cup of powdered clay into a selected liquid, such as distilled water or apple cider vinegar, then add 5 drops of pure EO per 1/4 cup of clay.<br><br>Apply clay mixture to desired area, allow to dry, then rinse or sponge off thoroughly with water (do not use soap). Complete the treatment with an application of body oil or lotion. |
| Steam Facial or Inhalation | Place 5 to 10 drops of EO into a bowl of hot water.<br><br>Place your face over the steaming bowl, covering your head with a towel. Remember to keep your eyes closed to avoid irritation from EO. Steam your face at a comfortable distance from the bowl until the water cools. Then rinse face with fresh cool water. |
| Body Lotion | For full body application, add 15 to 20 drops of pure EO to each 1 ounce of unscented (vegetable source) base lotion. |
| Skin Tonic Spritzer | Mix 4 ounces of distilled water with 20 to 30 drops of pure EO. Shake well before each use. Avoid spraying directly into eyes. Keep spritzer refrigerated to enhance its refreshing effect. |
| Air Freshener Spritzer | Mix 4 ounces of distilled water with 40 to 60 drops of pure EO. Shake well before each use. |

# Chakra Oil Blending Guide

Blend approximately 20 to 30 drops of combined essential oils to each 1/2 ounce of jojoba oil. For correct essential oil proportions, we suggest consulting an experienced aromatherapy practitioner. *These oils are intended for external use only.*

| CHAKRA | COLORS | ESSENTIAL OILS | STONES |
|---|---|---|---|
| #7 Crown | Violet | Angelica<br>Frankincense<br>Rosewood | Amethyst<br>Crystal |
| #6 Third eye | Indigo | Rosemary<br>Clary sage<br>Lavender | Lapis<br>Azurite |
| #5 Throat | Blue | Roman chamomile<br>Sandalwood<br>Myrrh | Turquoise<br>Blue lace agate |
| #4 Heart | Pink/Green | Geranium<br>Rose<br>Bergamot | Malachite<br>Rose quartz |
| #3 Solar/Spleen | Yellow | Neroli<br>Mandarin<br>Lemon<br>Grapefruit | Citrine<br>Amber |
| #2 Navel/Sacral | Orange | Jasmine (Absol)<br>Ginger<br>Sandalwood<br>Juniper<br>Sage | Carnelian<br>Gold topaz |
| #1 Base/Root | Red | Frankincense<br>Rosewood<br>Myrrh<br>Ylang Ylang<br>Vetiver | Garnet<br>Red jasper |

# Essential Oil Quick
# Reference Table

| ESSENTIAL OIL | PROPERTIES | CHARACTER | USES | METHODS |
|---|---|---|---|---|
| ANGELICA<br>*Angelica archangelica*<br>Roots | stomachic<br>anti-infectious<br>sudorific | purifying<br>restorative<br>protective | digestive aid<br>skin care<br>fragrance | massage<br>bath<br>compress |
| BASIL, exotic<br>*Ocimum basilicum*<br>Leaves | carminative<br>nervine<br>antispasmodic | revivifying<br>restorative<br>antidepressant | psychosomatic<br>gastrointestinal<br>respiratory | massage<br>inhalation<br>spritzer |
| BAY<br>*Pimenta racemosa*<br>Leaves | rubefacient<br>analgesic<br>decongestant | calming<br>relaxing | hair and scalp<br>insect repellent<br>respiratory | liniment<br>salve<br>massage |
| BAY LAUREL<br>*Laurus nobilis*<br>Leaves | carminative<br>bactericidal<br>hypotensive | restorative<br>sedative<br>antihysteric | digestive aid<br>fragrance<br>insect repellent | liniment<br>massage<br>salve |
| BERGAMOT<br>*Citrus bergamia*<br>Peel | antiseptic<br>antispasmodic<br>deodorant | calming<br>refreshing<br>antidepressant | skin care<br>anxiety<br>melancholia | diffusor, spritzer<br>bath<br>massage, compress |
| CARDAMOM<br>*Elletaria cardamomum*<br>Fruit | stomachic<br>deodorant<br>nervine | stimulant<br>brightening | digestive<br>halitosis<br>sciatica | mouthwash<br>topical |
| CARROT SEED<br>*Daucus carota*<br>Seeds | hepatic<br>depurative<br>diuretic | relaxing | skin care<br>genito-urinary<br>arthritis, rheumatism | massage<br>dermatology |

| Oil | Properties | Effects | Uses | Application |
|---|---|---|---|---|
| CEDARWOOD<br>*Cedrus atlanticus*<br>Wood | astringent<br>antispasmodic<br>antiseptic | protective<br>calming<br>grounding | insecticide<br>scalp care<br>fragrance | spritzer<br>skin care<br>massage |
| GERMAN CHAMOMILE<br>*Matricaria chamomilla*<br>Flower | anti-inflammatory<br>immunostimulant<br>antipyretic | calming<br>soothing | skin care<br>hair care | facial<br>bath<br>compress |
| ROMAN CHAMOMILE<br>*Anthemis nobilis*<br>Flower | anti-inflammatory<br>nervine<br>analgesic | sedative<br>antidepressant<br>restorative | body pain<br>hair care<br>skin care | massage<br>liniment<br>bath |
| CINNAMON<br>*Cinnamomum zeylanicum*<br>Bark | antiseptic<br>vermifuge<br>stomachic | warming<br>stimulating | scalp and skin care<br>fragrance<br>digestive | topical<br>foot massage |
| CLARY SAGE<br>*Salvia sclarea*<br>Leaves | antispasmodic<br>nervine | sedative<br>relaxant<br>euphoric | body care<br>menstrual<br>headache | massage<br>compress<br>bath |
| CLOVE BUD<br>*Eugenia caryophyllata*<br>Buds | parasiticidal<br>analgesic<br>antimicrobial | fortifying<br>clarifying<br>arousing | genito-urinary<br>respiratory<br>digestive | spritzer<br>dentifrice |
| CYPRESS<br>*Cupressus sempervirens*<br>Needles | styptic<br>deodorant<br>vasoconstrictive | soothing<br>relaxing | vascular<br>gynecologic<br>skin care | sitz bath<br>compress |
| ELEMI<br>*Canarium luzonicum*<br>Gum/resin | antiseptic<br>expectorant<br>tonic | rejuvenating<br>stimulating<br>fortifying | skin care<br>fragrance | spritzer<br>massage<br>inhalation |

| ESSENTIAL OIL | PROPERTIES | CHARACTER | USES | METHODS |
|---|---|---|---|---|
| EUCALYPTUS<br>*E. citriodora*<br>Leaves | anti-inflammatory<br>germicidal<br>decongestant | sedative<br>soothing<br>(lemony scent) | skin care<br>disinfectant<br>insect repellent | compress<br>bath<br>spritzer |
| EUCALYPTUS<br>*E. globulus*<br>Leaves | analgesic<br>bactericidal<br>expectorant | expansive<br>invigorating<br>(camphorous scent) | respiratory<br>rheumatism<br>insecticide | diffusor<br>massage<br>sauna, bath |
| EVERLASTING<br>*Helichrysum italicum*<br>Flowers | lymphatic<br>depurative<br>antiseptic | antidepressant<br>soothing | skin wounds<br>neuralgia<br>skin care | compress<br>massage |
| FENNEL<br>*Foeniculum vulgare*<br>Seeds/Roots/Leaves | carminative<br>laxative<br>diuretic | strengthening<br>encouraging | hair care<br>dieting<br>digestion | bath<br>compress<br>cellulite massage |
| FIR<br>*Abies siberica*<br>Needles | disinfectant<br>expectorant<br>deodorant | bracing<br>invigorating<br>energizing | respiratory<br>deodorant | diffusor, spritzer<br>sauna<br>back massage |
| FRANKINCENSE<br>*Boswellia carteri*<br>Resin | expectorant<br>antiseptic<br>cytophylactic | tranquilizing<br>meditative<br>protective | genito-urinary<br>skin treatment<br>fragrance | inhalation<br>massage<br>spritzer |
| GERANIUM<br>*Pelargonium graveolens*<br>Leaves | antiseptic<br>astringent<br>diuretic | balancing<br>stabilizing<br>antidepressant | fragrance<br>skin care<br>oral treatment | massage<br>facials<br>bath |

| Oil | Properties | Effects | Uses | Application |
|---|---|---|---|---|
| **GINGER** *Zingiber officinale* Roots | antiseptic, febrifuge, analgesic | fortifying, stimulative, aphrodisiac | cold treatment, body pain, digestive | liniment, compress, massage |
| **GRAPEFRUIT** *Citrus paradisi* Peel | hepatic, astringent, tonic | refreshing, uplifting | weight loss, digestive aid, oily skin care | diffusor, spritzer, massage |
| **JASMINE (absolute)** *Jasminum officinale* Flower | tonic, antispasmodic, nervine | euphoric, antidepressant, aphrodisiac | skin care, fragrance, psychotherapy | inhalation, massage, bath |
| **JUNIPER** *Juniperus communis* Fruit | diuretic, disinfectant, tonic | refreshing, stimulating | urinary, circulatory | massage, diffusor, spritzer, compress |
| **LAVENDER** *Lavandula officinalis* Flower | antiseptic, analgesic, anti-inflammatory | restorative, relaxing, cooling | skin care, respiratory, headache | massage, inhalation, bath, diffusor |
| **LEMON** *Citrus limonum* Peel | diuretic, stomachic, antiseptic | refreshing, reviving | skin care, circulatory, dyspepsia | massage, diffusor, spritzer, compress |
| **LEMONGRASS** *Andropogon citratus* Grass | deodorant, nervine, astringent | toning, refreshing, antidepressant | skin cleansing, disinfectant, foot care | massage, fragrance, aerosol, vaporization |
| **MANDARIN** *Citrus reticulata* Peel | antispasmodic, tonic, hypotensive | relaxing, heartening, antidepressant | fragrance, skin care, gastrointestinal | spritzer, bath, massage |

| ESSENTIAL OIL | PROPERTIES | CHARACTER | USES | METHODS |
|---|---|---|---|---|
| MARJORAM, FR. *Marjorana hortensis* Flower | antimicrobial laxative antispasmodic | anaphrodisiac tranquilizing restful | weight loss cramps fragrance | massage compress bath |
| MYRRH *Commiphora myrrha* Resin | preservative antiseptic anticatarrhal | fortifying sedative cooling | skin care dentifrice OB/GYN | inhalation wash massage |
| NEROLI (Orange Blossom) *Citrus aurantium* var. *amara* Flower | antispasmodic hypotensive germicidal | antidepressant restful aphrodisiac | fragrance skin care cardiovascular | massage bath inhalation |
| NIAOULI *Melaleuca viridiflora* Twigs/Leaves | anti-infectious vermifuge | balancing stimulating energizing | respiratory fatigue | massage inhalation |
| ORANGE *Citrus sinensis* Peel | anti-inflammatory hypotensive tonic | antidepressant soothing refreshing | oily skin care fragrance | spritzer inhalation |
| PALMAROSA *Cymbopogon martini* Leaves | hydrating tonic cytophylactic | clarifying refreshing | skin care fragrance | spritzer compress massage |
| PATCHOULI *Pogostemon cablin* Leaves | fungicidal cytophylactic anti-inflammatory | arousing aphrodisiac | skin and scalp care fragrance bites, stings | bath, compress spritzer massage |

| | | | | |
|---|---|---|---|---|
| PEPPER, BLACK<br>*Piper nigrum*<br>Fruit | antitoxin<br>analgesic<br>rubefacient | fortifying<br>strengthening | congestion<br>pain<br>rigidity | massage<br>bath<br>compress |
| PEPPERMINT<br>*Mentha piperita*<br>Leaves | analgesic<br>stomachic<br>decongestant | toning<br>invigorating<br>refreshing | digestive<br>respiratory<br>neuralgia | sauna, steam<br>inhalation<br>massage |
| PETITGRAIN (Orange Leaf)<br>*Citrus aurantium* var. *amara*<br>Leaves | nervine<br>antiperspirant<br>astringent | refreshing<br>clarifying<br>uplifting | skin care<br>hair care<br>fragrance | bath<br>massage<br>inhalation |
| PINE<br>*Pinus sylvestris*<br>Needles | disinfectant<br>expectorant<br>antiseptic | bracing<br>strengthening<br>stabilizing | respiratory<br>deodorant<br>genito-urinary | diffusor, spritzer<br>sauna<br>massage |
| ROSE<br>*Rose damascena*<br>Flower | antiseptic<br>anti-inflammatory<br>regulative | purifying<br>euphoric | skin care<br>fragrance<br>OB/GYN | massage<br>inhalation<br>bath |
| ROSEMARY<br>*Rosmarinus officinalis*<br>Leaves | nervine<br>antiseptic<br>analgesic | energizing<br>uplifting<br>stimulating | skin and hair care<br>biliousness<br>respiratory | bath<br>massage<br>diffusor, spritzer |
| ROSEWOOD (Bois de Rose)<br>*Aniba rosaeodora*<br>Wood | regulative<br>antibacterial<br>cytophylactic | euphoric<br>aphrodisiac<br>calming | fragrance<br>deodorant<br>skin care | bath<br>spritzer<br>massage |
| SANDALWOOD<br>*Santalum album*<br>Wood | diuretic<br>antiseptic<br>astringent | euphoric<br>grounding<br>aphrodisiac | skin care<br>fragrance<br>genito-urinary | massage<br>compress<br>sitz bath |

| ESSENTIAL OIL | PROPERTIES | CHARACTER | USES | METHODS |
|---|---|---|---|---|
| SPEARMINT *Mentha viridis* Leaves | tonic nervine stomachic | invigorating refreshing | digestive skin care fragrance | spritzer massage |
| SPIKE LAVENDER *Lavandula spica* Flower | antiseptic analgesic rubefacient | antidepressant tranquilizing | scalp and skin care insect repellent fragrance | sport massage bath inhalation |
| SPIKENARD *Aralia racemosa* Root | tonic diuretic analgesic | stimulating restorative | skin care pulmonary OB/GYN | massage compress bath |
| SPRUCE, BLACK *Picea mariana* Needles | expectorant tonic analgesic | bracing revitalizing steadying | respiratory genito-urinary body pain | massage inhalation compress |
| TEA TREE *Melaleuca alternifolia* Leaves | fungicidal antimicrobial parasiticidal | cooling balsamic | disinfectant scalp and skin care oral hygiene | bath diffusor massage |
| VETIVER *Andropogon muricatus* Roots | rubefacient hydrating | grounding steadying | psychologic fragrance mature skin care | lotions bath massage |
| YARROW *Achillea millefolium* Flowers | anti-inflammatory styptic hypotensive | balancing soothing | skin care hair care cardiovascular | massage inhalation compress |
| YLANG YLANG *Cananga odorata* Flower | hypotensive hydrating regulative | aphrodisiac sedative antidepressant | skin care cardiopulmonary fragrance | massage bath diffusor, spritzer |

# Essential Oil Repertory

*Important Reminder:* This repertory is a general reference only. Consult Chapter 7, "Essential Oil Profiles" and other chapters for more specific information about the properties and uses of the essential oils listed in each category before making selections for any condition.

## Abrasions

lavender, sandalwood, yarrow

## Acne

bergamot, chamomile (Roman), clove, everlasting, juniper, lavender, lemongrass, petitgrain, rosemary, yarrow

## Anxiety

basil, bergamot, cedarwood, chamomile (Roman), cypress, geranium, jasmine, juniper, lavender, marjoram (French), neroli, petitgrain, rose, ylang ylang

## Apathy

jasmine, juniper, patchouli, peppermint

## Appetite

angelica, bergamot, fennel, ginger, black pepper, vetiver

## Arthritis

angelica, carrot seed, frankincense, ginger, juniper, vetiver

## Asthma

basil, clary sage, clove, black spruce

## Athlete's Foot

bay laurel, clove, lavender, lemongrass, myrrh, patchouli, tea tree

## Bloating

mandarin, marjoram (French), rosemary

## Body Odor

bergamot, clary sage, cypress, lavender, lemongrass, neroli, petitgrain, rosewood

## Boils (Abscess)

carrot seed, chamomile (Roman), spike lavender, spikenard, tea tree

## Bruises

bay laurel, chamomile (German or Roman), everlasting, lavender, marjoram (French)

## Burns

chamomile (Roman), everlasting, geranium, lavender, niaouli, rosemary, spike lavender

## Cellulite

cypress, fennel, geranium, ginger, grapefruit, juniper, lemon, black pepper, rosemary

## Circulatory

angelica, carrot seed, chamomile (Roman), garlic, lemon, neroli, black pepper, peppermint, rose, rosemary, spikenard, black spruce, yarrow, ylang ylang

## Colic

bergamot, chamomile (Roman), fennel, juniper, neroli, peppermint

## Constipation

fennel, ginger, mandarin, marjoram (French), rose, rosemary

## Cough

cypress, eucalyptus, everlasting, ginger, jasmine, juniper, black spruce

## Cramps

chamomile (Roman), geranium, mandarin, neroli, peppermint, rosemary

## Depression

basil, bergamot, chamomile (Roman), clary sage, frankincense, geranium, grapefruit, jasmine, lavender, lemon, mandarin, neroli, orange, sandalwood, ylang ylang

## Dermatitis

carrot seed, chamomile (Roman), patchouli, rosemary

## Despair

angelica, rose

## Diabetes

cinnamon, eucalyptus, geranium

## Diarrhea

cardamom, clove, cypress, frankincense, ginger, myrrh, neroli, black pepper

## Dyspepsia

angelica, basil, bergamot, chamomile (Roman), cardamom, clary sage, clove, fennel, lemon, mandarin, black pepper, peppermint, petitgrain

## Ear

chamomile (Roman), fennel, lavender, tea tree

## Eczema

carrot seed, chamomile (German), everlasting, fennel, myrrh, patchouli, petitgrain, rose, rosemary

## Edema

cardamom, carrot seed, clove, grapefruit, juniper, lemon, lemongrass, patchouli, black pepper, rosemary, sandalwood, spikenard

## Fainting

basil, peppermint

## Fatigue

basil, everlasting, geranium, lavender, peppermint, rosemary

## Fever

chamomile (German or Roman), clove, ginger, lemon, lemongrass, peppermint, yarrow

## Flatulence

angelica, bergamot, cardamom, clary sage, ginger, marjoram (French), black pepper, peppermint, rosemary

## Gallbladder

chamomile (Roman), grapefruit, lemon, rose, rosemary

## Gastric

angelica, basil, bay laurel, bergamot, cardamom, chamomile (German), clove, fennel, ginger, grapefruit, lemon, lemongrass, mandarin, black pepper, peppermint, petitgrain

## Gout

angelica, carrot seed, chamomile (German or Roman), clove, fennel, garlic, juniper

## Grief

marjoram (French), neroli, rose

## Hair (Scalp)

bay, clary sage, clove, geranium, lavender, palmarosa, patchouli, petitgrain, rosemary, tea tree, yarrow, ylang ylang

## Headache

clary sage, ginger, lavender, lemongrass, peppermint, rosemary, rosewood

## Heart

lavender, mandarin, neroli, ylang ylang

## Herpes

geranium, lavender, tea tree

## Hiccough

angelica, fennel, mandarin

## Hostility

chamomile (Roman), cypress, lavender, marjoram (French), ylang ylang

## Hypertension

clary sage, garlic, juniper, lavender, mandarin, yarrow, ylang ylang

## Hypotension

garlic, ginger, black pepper, rosemary

## Hysteria

bay laurel, chamomile (Roman), clary sage, lavender, ylang ylang

## Influenza (Colds and Flu)

angelica, cinnamon, cypress, eucalyptus, garlic, geranium, ginger, lavender, myrrh, black pepper, peppermint, pine, tea tree

## Insect Bites and Stings

basil, eucalyptus, geranium, lavender, lemon, patchouli, rosemary, tea tree

## Kidney

carrot seed, chamomile (German), fennel, juniper, lemon

## Liver

carrot seed, chamomile (German or Roman), everlasting, fennel, grapefruit, mandarin, rose, rosemary

## Menstrual

basil, bay laurel, carrot seed, chamomile (German or Roman), clary sage, cypress, fennel, geranium, jasmine, lavender, myrrh, yarrow

## Migraine

basil, chamomile (Roman), eucalyptus, everlasting, lavender, marjoram (French)

## Muscular-Skeletal Aches and Pains

bay, chamomile (German or Roman), eucalyptus, ginger, lavender, lemongrass, marjoram (French), black pepper, peppermint, pine, rosemary, black spruce

## Nausea

basil, cardamom, chamomile (Roman), fennel, ginger, lavender, mandarin, black pepper, peppermint, rosewood

## Nerves

angelica, basil, bay, cardamom, clary sage, everlasting, geranium, juniper, lavender, neroli, rosemary, vetiver

## Neuralgia

bay, chamomile (Roman), everlasting, peppermint

## Oral

cardamom, chamomile (Roman), clove, fennel, geranium, lemon, myrrh, niaouli, peppermint, tea tree

## Panic

clary sage, jasmine, lavender, neroli

## Paranoia

basil, clary sage, frankincense, jasmine, juniper

## Parasites

bergamot, clove, eucalyptus, fennel, frankincense, garlic, lemon, lemongrass, myrrh, peppermint, rosemary, tea tree

## PMS

carrot seed, chamomile (Roman), clary sage, fennel, geranium, neroli, patchouli, yarrow, ylang ylang

## Psoriasis

carrot seed, everlasting, myrrh

## Rash

angelica, carrot seed, chamomile (Roman), lavender, sandalwood, yarrow

## Respiratory

angelica, basil, bay, clove, eucalyptus, fir, frankincense, jasmine, lavender, lemon, marjoram (French), myrrh, niaouli, peppermint, pine, rosemary, sandalwood, black spruce, tea tree

## Rheumatism

angelica, bay, bay laurel, carrot seed, chamomile (Roman), eucalyptus, frankincense, ginger, juniper, lavender, spikenard, black spruce

## Sexual

clary sage, clove, ginger, jasmine, marjoram (French), neroli, patchouli, rose, rosewood, sandalwood, ylang ylang

## Sinus

basil, eucalyptus, lavender, peppermint, pine, tea tree

## Skin

| | |
|---|---|
| *Dry:* | everlasting, frankincense, geranium, jasmine, neroli, palmarosa, patchouli, rose, rosemary, vetiver, ylang ylang |
| *Oily:* | bergamot, chamomile (Roman), clary sage, cypress, everlasting, geranium, juniper, lemon, lemongrass, myrrh, niaouli, rosemary, yarrow, ylang ylang |
| *Puffy:* | cypress, juniper, lavender, lemon, lemongrass, petitgrain |
| *Sensitive:* | chamomile (German or Roman), clary sage, lavender, neroli, rose, sandalwood, yarrow |
| *Wrinkled:* | carrot seed, everlasting, frankincense, geranium, jasmine, juniper, lemon, myrrh, palmarosa, patchouli, rose, rosemary, rosewood, sandalwood, vetiver, ylang ylang |

## Sleep

basil, chamomile (Roman), clary sage, everlasting, lavender, mandarin, marjoram (French), neroli, sandalwood, ylang ylang

## Sores (Ulcers)

carrot seed, chamomile (German), everlasting, frankincense, geranium, myrrh, niaouli, yarrow

## Throat

clary sage, eucalyptus, geranium, jasmine, myrrh, black pepper, sandalwood, tea tree

## Toothache

chamomile (Roman), clove, black pepper, peppermint

## Uncertainty

angelica, basil, cypress, juniper, patchouli, rosemary, rosewood

## Urinary

bergamot, carrot seed, chamomile (German), clove, fennel, frankincense, juniper, lemon, patchouli, pine, rosemary, sandalwood, black spruce, tea tree

## Vaginal

geranium, lavender, myrrh, niaouli, rose, spikenard, tea tree

## Varicosity

cypress, frankincense, juniper, lemongrass, myrrh, neroli, sandalwood, spikenard, yarrow

## Vertigo (Dizziness)

basil, chamomile (Roman), clary sage, clove, lavender, peppermint

## Wounds

carrot seed, chamomile (German), clove, everlasting, frankincense, geranium, lavender, myrrh, niaouli, patchouli, yarrow

# Selected Bibliography

Chishti, Hakim M., N.D. *Natural Medicine: The Herbal Therapeutics of Avicenna.* New York: McGraw Hill, 1979.

Gattefossé, René-Maurice. *Aromathérapie.* Paris: Giradot & Cie, 1937.

———. *Gattefossé's Aromatherapy.* Saffron Walden Essex: C.W. Daniel, 1993.

Gruner, O. Cameron, M.D. *A Treatise on the Canon of Medicine of Avicenna.* New York: Augustus M. Kelley, 1979.

Guenther, Ernest, Ph.D. *The Essential Oils.* 6 vol. Malabar, FL: Robert E. Krieger, 1972–85.

Gümbel, Dietrich, Ph.D. *Principles of Holistic Therapy with Herbal Essences.* Heidelberg: Karl F. Haug, 1986.

Lautié, Raymond, D.Sc. and André Passebecq, M.D. *Aromatherapy: The Use of Plant Essences in Healing.* Wellingborough Northhamptonshire: Thorsons, 1984.

Lavabre, Marcel. *Aromatherapy Workbook.* Rochester, VT: Healing Arts, 1990.

Maury, Marguerite. *The Secret of Life and Youth.* London: Macdonald, 1964.

Shook, Edward E., M.D. *Advanced Treatise in Herbology.* Beaumont, CA: Trinity Center, 1978.

———. *Elementary Treatise in Herbology.* Beaumont, CA: Trinity Center, 1974.

Thomas, Lewis. *The Lives of a Cell.* New York: Viking, 1974.

Tisserand, Robert. *Aromatherapy to Heal and Tend the Body.* Santa Fe, NM: Lotus, 1988.

———. *The Art of Aromatherapy.* Rochester, VT: Inner Traditions, 1979.

————. *The Essential Oil Safety Data Manual.* Brighton Sussex: Association of Tisserand Aromatherapists, 1985.

Valnet, Jean, M.D. *The Practice of Aromatherapy.* Rochester, VT: Destiny Books, 1982.

Van Toller, Steve and George H. Dodd, eds. *Perfumery: The Psychology and Biology of Fragrance.* London: Chapman & Hall, 1988.

# Aromatherapy Essential Oil Companies

Aroma Vera
5901 Rodeo Road
Los Angeles, CA 90016
(800) 669-9514

Original Swiss Aromatics
P.O. Box 6842
San Rafael, CA 94903
(415) 459-3998

Time Laboratories
P.O. Box 3243
South Pasadena, CA 91031
(818) 300-8096

Tisserand Aromatherapy
P.O. Box 750428
Petaluma, CA 94975
(707) 769-5120

Windrose Aromatics, Inc.
12629 North Tatum Boulevard
Suite 611
Phoenix, AZ 85032
(602) 992-5390

# Index

abrasions, 223

*absolutes,* 2

acne, 223

adrenal glands, 143, 145–146, 147

affinity, principle of, 164

After-Flight Regulator blends, 109

aguesia, 67

air freshener spritzer, 212

air quality, 112–113

alcohol, in perfumery, 24–25

allopathy, 33–34

*Al-Qanum fi'l Tibb (The Canon of Medicine)* (Avicenna), 7

alternative therapies, 3-4, 33–35, 121-122, 123-126

ambient fragrancing. *See* environmental fragrancing

American Medical Association, 121

angelica, 147, 179–180, 213, 216

anise, 171

anosmia, 67, 68

antibiotics, vs. essential oils, 13–14

antioxidants, 50

anxiety, 150, 223

apathy, 223

appetite, 223

Arabs, 5–6

Arcier, Micheline, 12

"aroma-chology," 119–121

aromapsychology, 5. *See also* emotions, psyche, psychology

aromatherapy, 1, 11–12, 23–24

vs. "aroma-chology," 119–121

vs. aromatics, 3, 19

in athletics, 108–109

in big business, 16

in Europe, 126–128

vs. fragrance industry, 152–153

medical politics and, 121–126

vs. phytotherapy, 3

for women, 39–42, 105

*See also* phytoaromatherapy

aromatics, 3–12, 21

vs. aromatherapy, 3, 19

aromatogram, 45–48

arthritis, 224

Asclepiades, 5

astral body, 150

athlete's foot, 224

athletics, 108–109

asthma, 224
aura, 160
aversion therapy, 151–153
Avicenna, 6–7
Ayurvedic medicine, 3–4

base note, 26
basil, 155, 180–181, 216
baths, 211
bay, 181–182, 216
bay laurel, 216
behavioral modification, 140
Belaiche, Paul, 12
bergamot, 150, 182
bloating, 224
body lotion, 212
body odor, 224
body oil, 211
body pack, clay, 212
boils, 224
boldo, 41
brain
    chemistry of, 90–92
    hemispheres of, 76–78, 148–150
    olfaction and, 74–83
    PET scanning of, 157–159
    See also memory, mind
Broca, Paul, 74
bruises, 224
Brunschweig, Hieronymous, 8
burns, 224

cacosmia, 67
Caesar, Julius, 21
Cajola, Renato, 11
calamus, 41
camphor, 171
carbon dioxide extraction, 176–178
cardamom, 183, 216
carrot seed, 183–184, 216

Cayola, Renato, 150
cedarwood, 217
cellulite, 224
central nervous system, 78–79
cerebrum, 76
chakra oil blending guide, 213
chamomile
    German, 45, 184, 217
    Roman, 184–185, 213, 217
Charles II, King (England), 23
"chemically hypersensitive," 110–111
chemical solvents, 2
chemotypes, 167–169
China, 3, 4, 15
chromatography, 173–175
cinchona, 134
cinnamon, 45, 171, 217
circulatory problems, 225
clary sage, 150, 185–186, 213, 217
clove, 45, 50, 186–187, 217
coca, 136
cognition, and olfaction, 83–85, 89–90,
    94, 142
colds, 228
colic, 225
concrétes, 2
conditioned reflex, 151
consciousness, 134–137, 159
constipation, 225
cortisone, 146
cosmetology, 15–16
cough, 225
Couvreur, Albert, 11
cramps, 225
Culpeper, Nicholas, 8
culture, and olfaction, 73–74
cypress, 150, 187–188, 217

Davis, Patricia, 12, 40
decoction, 3

depression, 150, 225
dermatitis, 225
despair, 225
diabetes, 225
diarrhea, 226
diffusors, 209–210, 211
Dioscorides, 5
disease, theories of, 9–10, 34–35
distillation, 6, 7–8
    steam, 1, 24–25, 176
dizziness, 232
Dodd, George, 127
"dominose effect," 61–62
Douek, E., 68
drugs, 8–9, 14, 24
    vs. essential oils, 37–38
    synthetic steroids, 146–147
*Dynamic Neuroscience: Its Application
    to Brain Disorders* (Watts), 75
dysguesia, 67
dysosmia, 67, 69, 70
dyspepsia, 226

ear, 226
eczema, 226
edema, 226
Egypt, 3, 4, 20–21
elemi, 217
Elizabeth I, Queen (England), 22
endocrine glands, 143, 145–146
environmental fragrancing, 22, 109–119,
    137–139
emotions, 5, 83–85, 90–92, 96–100.
    *See also* psyche, psychology
essential oils
    affinity principle and, 164–165
    antimicrobial properties of, 10,
        13–14, 44–48, 168–169
    antioxidant properties of, 50
    blending, 210

chemical analysis of, 173–175
in cosmetology, 15–16
vs. drugs, 37–38
electrochemical properties of, 48–50
electromagnetic properties of, 18
empirical evidence about, 36–37
etheric nature of, 162–163
extraction of, 1–2, 8, 176–178
food industry use of, 4
hazardous, 41–42
in homeostasis, 35
hormonal effects of, 145
laboratory experiments on, 36–37,
    45–48
natural vs. synthetic, 16, 86–87,
    88, 92, 130–132, 137, 138–140,
    149
pure, 1–2
psycho-physiological effects of,
    17–19, 55, 131–132, 141–143,
    149–150
in psychotherapy, 150–153
safety of, 38–39, 169–173
skin absorption of, 42–44
therapeutic effects of, 10, 13–14,
    51–54
vibrational energies of, 18
*See also* synthetic oils
ether (life energy), 53–54, 162–163
etheric double, 160, 161
eucalyptus, 188, 218
Europe, 7–10, 22–23, 126–128
everlasting, 188–189, 218

facial application, 211, 212
fainting, 226
fatigue, 226
Federal Trade Commission, 121–122
fennel, 171, 189–190, 218
fever, 226

fir, 218
fish-odor syndrome, 70
flatulence, 227
floral waters, 6, 209
flu, 228
Food and Drug Administration, 122, 172
food industry, essential oils in, 4
fragrance, 19–25, 28–32
    synthetic, 120–121, 130–132
    *See also* perfumery
Fragrance Foundation, 119–121
fragrance industry, 122–123, 125, 152–153
Fragrance Research Fund, 89, 118–119
Franchomme, Pierre, 12, 167
frankincense, 190–191, 213, 218
free radicals, 50
Freud, Sigmund, 69, 152

gallbladder, 227
garlic, 51
gastric problems, 227
Gattefossé, René-Maurice, 11
Gatti, Giovanni, 11, 150
gender, and olfaction, 101–105
George III, King (England), 23
geranium, 147, 191, 213, 218
Gerard, John, 8
ginger, 191–192, 213, 219
Girault, Dr. Maurice, 45–46
gout, 227
grapefruit, 192, 213, 219
Greece, 5–6, 21–22
grief, 227
Gümbel, Dr. Dietrich, 43–44
gustation, 67, 70, 71

hair, 227
Hatshepsut, Queen, 20

headache, 227
heart, 227
heliotropin, 87
herbalism, 3
herpes, 227
hiccough, 228
hippocampus, 75, 156–157
Hippocrates, 5
holistic healing, 33–35
homeostasis, 35, 51
hormones, 143–148
horseradish, 41
hostility, 228
hyperosmia, 67, 72
hypertension, 228
hypoguesia, 67
hypotension, 228
hypothalamus, 75
hyssop, 41, 171
hysteria, 228

immunology, and olfaction, 65–67
India, 3, 15, 21
infection, 10, 13–14, 44–48, 168–169
influenza, 228
infusion, 3
inhalation, 211
insect bites and stings, 228
intelligence, 162
International Flavors and Fragrances, 128

James, William, 97, 159
Japan, 109–110, 114–115
jasmine, 86–87, 141–143, 150, 192–193, 213, 219
juniper, 39, 193–194, 213, 219

ketones, 171
kidney, 228

Kirlian effect, 53

laboratory science, and phytoaroma-
    therapy, 36–37, 45–48
Lapraz, Jean-Claude, 12, 47, 168
lavender, 11, 16, 141–143, 150, 195–195,
    213, 219
"Law of All or Nothing," 168–169
learning, 151–153, 155
left brain, 77–78, 148
legislation
    alternative therapies, 121–122, 125
    environmental fragrancing, 110–112
lemon, 45, 84, 150, 195–196, 213, 219
lemongrass, 45, 219
lemon verbena, 150
Lily, Charles, 23
limbic system, 74–76, 155–157
lime, 150
liniments, 3
liver, 228
Lives of a Cell (Thomas), 57
Louis XI, King, 69
Louis XIV, King, 23

mandarin, 196, 213, 219
marjoram, 150, 197, 220
massage, aromatic, 4, 15, 211
Maury, Marguerite, 11–12, 138
medical politics, aromatherapy and,
    121–126
medicinal plants, 132–138
medicine
    essential oils in, 13–14
    Ayurvedic, 3–4
Médicis, Catherine de, 22
melissa, 171
memory, 153–160
    See also brain, mind
menstrual problems, 229

mental disorders, and olfaction, 69
Mesopotamia, 4
Middle East, 4–6
middle note, 26
migraine, 229
mind, 89–90, 161–162
    See also psyche
Monell Chemical Senses Center, 113,
    118
mood. See emotions
mouth, 229
muguet, 92
mugwort, 41, 171, 173
muscular-skeletal aches and pains, 229
musk, 142, 149
mustard, 41, 171
myrrh, 197–198, 213, 220

naturopathy, 33–35
nausea, 229
Nero, Claudius, 21
neroli, 150, 198–199, 213, 220
nervousness, 229
neuralgia, 229
neurotransmitters, 144
niaouli, 199, 220
noradrenaline, 145
nose, 56–60
nostril cycle, 80–81

obstetrics, aromatherapy in, 39–42
odors
    judgement and, 93–96
    memory and, 153–160
    perception of, 59–60
    performance and, 92–93
    personality and, 100–101, 105–107
    sexuality and, 62–65
    sleep and, 85–89
    subliminal influence of, 85

olfaction, 61–62
  brain and, 74–83
  emotions and, 83–85, 90–92, 96–100
  evolution of, 56–58
  gender differences in, 101–105
  immunology and, 65–67
  mental disorders and, 69
  nostril cycle, 80–81
  pheromones and, 62–65
  in pregnancy, 71–72
  psycho-physiological aspects of, 81–85
  research in, 17–19
olfactory communication, 72–74
olfactory system, 59–60
  nerves, 79–83
  vomeronasal organ, 63–65
oral problems, 229
orange, 150, 220
oregano, 171
osha, 134
osmatic, 67, 72
osmesis, 67
osmic frequencies, 60
osmology, 67–74
osphresis, 67

palmarosa, 199–100, 220
panic, 229
Papez-MacLean theory of limbic system, 155
Paracelsus, 8, 24
paranoia, 230
parasites, 230
Parkinson, John, 8
parosmia, 67
partial reinforcement, 151
patchouli, 200, 220
pennyroyal, 41, 171
Penoel, Daniel, 12

pepper, black, 200, 221
peppermint, 50, 86, 92, 155, 201, 221
performance, 92–93
perfume, 23, 25–28
perfumery, 23–25, 28–30
  vs. aromatics, 3
*Perfumery: The Psychology and Biology of Fragrance* (Van Toller & Dodd), 127
Persia, 3, 6
personality, scent and, 100–101, 105–107
perspiration, 43, 63, 65
petitgrain, 150, 201–202, 221
pharmaceutical industry, 9
pharmacology, vs. aromatherapy, 37–38
phenols, 171
pheromones, 62–65
Philip II, King (France), 22
phobias, 108
phytoaromatherapy, 35
  clinical, 44–48
  laboratory science and, 36–37
  vs. pharmacology, 37–38
  *See also* aromatherapy
phytohormones, 1
phytotherapy, 2–3
pine, 142, 147, 202, 221
plants
  medicinal, 132–138
  psychoactive, 134–137
Plato, 152
pleasure principle, 152
PMS, 230
positive reinforcement, 151–153
*Practice of Aromatherapy, The* (Valnet), 11, 13, 34, 42, 45, 46, 48
pregnancy
  aromatherapy in, 39–42
  olfaction in, 71–72

Price, Shirley, 12

primer pheromones, 64

*Principles of Holistic Therapy with Herbal Essences* (Gumbel), 43

psoriasis, 230

psyche, 160–162

  and olfaction, 81–85

  *See also* emotions, mind

psychology

  aromatics in, 5, 17–19, 141–143

  *See also* emotions, mind

*Psychology and Biology of Fragrance, The* (Douek), 68

psychopharmacology, 134–137

psychotherapy, 150–153

quinine, 134

rash, 230

respiratory problems, 230

retail industry, environmental fragrancing in, 116–118

rheumatism, 230

right brain, 77–78, 95, 148

Rome, 5–6, 21–22

rose, 16, 150, 202–203, 213, 221

rosemary, 147, 155, 171, 203–204, 213, 221

rosewood, 204, 213, 221

Rovesti, Dr. Paolo, 12, 50, 87, 150, 151

rue, 41

Ryman, Daniele, 12

sage, 39, 171, 213

  clary. *See* clary sage

sandalwood, 45, 150, 204–205, 213, 221

savin, 40, 41, 171

scalp, 227

scent. *See* odors

Schiffman, Dr. Susan, 68, 73–74, 118, 151

*Secret of Life and Youth, The* (Maury), 11–12

serotonin, 145, 147

sexuality, and odors, 62–65

sexual problems, 230

Shiseido, 115–116

"sick buildings," 129

signaling pheromones, 64

sinus problems, 231

skin, 42–44, 230, 231

skin tonic spritzer, 212

sleep, 231

smell. *See* olfaction

*soma*, 160–162

sores, 231

soul, 160–162

spearmint, 222

spectroscopy, 173–175

spike lavender, 222

spikenard, 205, 222

spirit, 161–162

spruce, black, 206, 222

steam distillation, 1, 24–25, 176

steroids, synthetic, 146–147

stimulus discrimination, 151

stimulus generalization, 151

synthetic oils, 3, 19, 86–87, 88, 92, 93

  *See also* essential oils

tansy, 41, 171

taste, 67, 70–71

tea tree, 11, 44, 206–207, 222

terpene, 166, 171–172

terrain, 47

Thatcher, Margaret, 127

Thomas, Lewis, 57

throat, 231

thuja, 42, 171
thyme, 39, 45, 147, 171
*thymos*, 160, 161
Tibb medicine, 7, 9
tinctures, 3
Tissarand, Maggie, 40
Tisserand, Robert, 12
toothache, 231
top note, 26
toxic essential oils, 41–42
trigeminal nerve, 59

uncertainty, 231
urinary problems, 232

vaginal problems, 232
Valnet, Dr. Jean, 9–10, 11, 13, 34, 42,
    45, 46, 48, 50, 168
vanillin, 84

Van Toller, Steve, 127
varicosity, 232
Vedas, aromatics mentioned in, 3
vetiver, 207, 213, 222
vertigo, 232
Villanova, Arnald de, 7
violet leaf, 150
vomeronasal organ, 63–65

Watts, G. O., 75
wintergreen, 42, 171
women, 103–105
wormseed, 42, 171
wormwood, 42, 171
Worwood, Valerie Ann, 40
wounds, 232

yarrow, 207–208, 222
ylang ylang, 150, 208, 213, 222